# Effective Technology Integration for Disabled Children

Malka Margalit

# Effective Technology Integration for Disabled Children

## The Family Perspective

Springer-Verlag
New York Heidelberg Berlin
London Paris Tokyo Hong Kong

Malka Margalit, Ph.D.
School of Education
Tel-Aviv University
Ramat-Aviv 69978, Israel

Library of Congress Cataloging-in-Publication Data
Margalit, Malka.
Effective technology integration for disabled children : the family perspective / Malka Margalit.
p. cm.
Includes bibliographical references (p. ).
1. Handicapped children – Education – Data processing.
2. Handicapped children – Education – Data processing – Case studies.
3. Computer-assisted instruction. I. Title.
LC4024.M37 1990 90-32519
317.9′043 – dc20

Printed on acid-free paper


Softcover reprint of the hardcover 1st edition 1990



Camera-ready copy provided by the author.

9 8 7 6 5 4 3 2 1

ISBN-13:978-1-4613-9008-4 e-ISBN-13:978-1-4613-9006-0
DOI: 10.1007/978-1-4613-9006-0

*To my family*

# Foreword

Research to determine the effects of microcomputer applications as compared to more traditional pedagogical approaches in the schools has been generally disappointing. When applied to differential effects with non-handicapped pupils the aggregate evidence suggests equivocal outcomes at best. The present writer's research and critical reviews of the empirical evidence for microcomputer effects with handicapped children has yielded similarly unconvincing conclusions. In fact, the lack of empirical evidence supports the contention that there is currently little or no objective justification for large scale adoption of computers to enhance the achievement of handicapped pupils in the schools. We now recognize that simply searching for main effects of machines on the academic and/or social achievement of school children is a naive endeavor which will probably continue to yield unproductive outcomes. It has become evident that computers are the "vehicles that deliver instruction but [they] do not influence student achievement any more than the truck that delivers our groceries causes changes in our nutrition" (Clark, 1983, p.445). Most empiricists recognize that until researchers study the effects of microcomputers interacting with relevant user, software, content and other social and instructional delivery variables, we probably will not succeed in understanding and/or maximizing the contributions of technological interventions in the education of disabled learners. There is a clear need for new and thoughtful conceptual models that consider the information processing characteristics of disabled learners in relationship to the delivery of effective mediating variables related to technology applications, and that have potential for enhancing the adaptive behavior of such users within specified content domains.

Why are educational administrators expending scarce financial resources to acquire microcomputers in the face of their uncertain educational effects? Why are parents impelled to purchase personal computers for their homes? Computer use in many contemporary societal contexts is being promoted to convey the connotation of educational competence and of the *avant garde*; and computer ownership has emerged as a significant status symbol within many important institutions in almost all societies. The allure and commercially driven promise of potentially powerful, but as yet unsubstantiated, educational effects of microcomputer applications has propelled a wide international market toward mass diffusion and adoption of these machines. People throughout the world are being attracted to computers by promotions in the mass media, through personal experiences with technology in the work place, and by observations of rapid transformations to automation in virtually all facets of their lives.

The "technology revolution" is widely perceived as having important implications for virtually all facets of our society. Parents of school children have come to expect much from the educational applications of microcomputers in the schools. Many parents believe their children must learn to be active computer users or they will be left behind and denied the fruits of a better future. Schools and families are being pressed to instruct all children to acquire computer literacy skills. The lack of ubiquitous scientific evidence for the much heralded expectations of computer assisted instruction (CAI) has not apparently constrained enthusiastic response for adoption of these innovations. Parents of disabled children with marked academic and social individual differences, are also demanding that their children become computer literate and socially identified as computer users.

Dr. Malka Margalit's critical analytic and empirical concerns with microcomputers, handicapped children and their families must be viewed within the context of a number of important foci. First, she recognizes that microcomputers studied alone are not apt to produce dramatic educational or social effects. The machines are not considered independent from other important dynamic social and educational variables that interact in conducting innovative interventions. Hence, she resists asking the simplistic and naive empirical questions about microcomputer effects that have previously produced unimpressive empirical results. She is obviously not interested in considering Clark's "delivery truck" in isolation -- but she does focus on the interaction between the vehicle, its contents, its context and its drivers. She is interested in the complexities associated with what the present writer has referred to elsewhere as *Micro-Educational Environments*

(Semmel & Lieber, 1986). Margalit knows that complex systems produce complex problems and answers. Accordingly, her focus breaks with much of the past research in the area by eschewing standard reductionistic experimental methodologies while favoring rational analysis, ethnographic and case study approaches which produce richer descriptions of her theoretical contributions, intervention processes and computer literacy effects.

Margalit's model characterizes the fundamental deficits of mildly retarded and learning disabled students as falling within an information processing paradigm. She sees particular deficits in speed or efficiency in processing information; these learners are deemed to have impoverished repertoires of previous learning (knowledge bases); they are presumed to be poor in acquisition strategies, memory and problem solving; and they are seen as poor in metacognitive functioning. She seeks to identify appropriate principles of learning within the context of her model toward realizing successful intervention of computerized activities within the home and school. Consistent with contemporary cognitive science theory, she sees the necessity for developing computer programs that train translation, schemata, strategy and automaticity skills. The computer is seen as a valuable tool for developing both general procedural and content specific knowledge through augmented home instruction. Margalit cautiously discusses the potential value of utilizing gaming, simulation, drill-and-practice, and word processing modes of computer presentation in the home toward reaching goals for the development of cognitive and metacognitive strategies among disabled students.

A unique focus of Margalit's work rests with her sensitivity to the broad psycho-social impact that the technology revolution is having on both disabled school children and their families. She understands the frustrating nature of parenting handicapped children in societies characterized by highly valuing academic achievement. Her unique contribution is precisely in her recognition of the unprecedented opportunities presented by the infusion of computers into the home. Her central thesis brings to our attention the potential facilitating role of the family in supporting the disabled child's home computing activities. Family dynamics are related to empowering parents to support their child's needs for computer competence. The analysis of the stresses impinging on families of handicapped students and the role of family climate on children's academic performance includes scholarly insights pertaining to father and mother roles in the family. Margalit understands that mothers are more vulnerable than fathers in regard to coping with the stress of rearing the disabled child in the family social matrix. Computers at home may enhance the child's personal growth, and also may promote a helping climate for the entire family. For example, the presence of the home computer might provide opportunities for a greater child rearing role for fathers which could result in a reduction of maternal stress within the family unit. Stress reduction, control of resources and development of coping strategies are associates of parent "empowerment" relative to intervening at home in actively pursuing the computer competency objectives established for disabled children. Hence, through these conceptualized family roles in enhancing and instructing instruction for handicapped children, Margalit envisions the computer as a new bridge between the school and the home.

Upon completion of this monograph, the reader will surely recognize that Malka Margalit's work is clearly not the product of a technological zealot. Rather, this scholarly text represents a significant theoretically driven effort by a special educator and socio-behavioral scientist who is interested in the human factors that are most likely to result in maximizing the use of technology to further the adaptive competence of handicapped learners and their families. Hence, this volume stands alone as a unique entry into the multifaceted dimensions of inquiry relating handicapped learners, their families and the supported intervention of microcomputer applications for the purpose of maximizing multiple educational and social outcomes. The text most assuredly will engage the reader's interest for its superb synthesis of empirical literature related to the topics explored and will foster a deeper level of analysis of these issues than has hitherto been experienced -- and will certainly stimulate and nurture a new line of needed programmatic research in this exciting new area of inquiry.

Melvyn I. Semmel, Professor & Director
Special Education Research Laboratory
University of California, Santa Barbara

**References**

Clark, R. E. (1983). Reconsidering research on learning from media. *Review of Educational Research*, *53*(4), 445-459.

Semmel, M. I., & Lieber, J. A. (1986). Computer applications in instruction. *Focus on Exceptional Children*, *18*(9), 1-12.

# Preface

The conceptualization of the stress, resources, and coping paradigm in families with mildly handicapped children has rapidly become the center of interest for research, clinical practice, and special education. In this volume, mildly handicapped children are referred to as a generic group including children with learning disabilities, mild mental retardation, and mild behavioral difficulties. The critical role that parents of these youngsters may play in fostering their children's development, which was acknowledged and demonstrated through extensive research, served as the impetus for this effort to identify effective intervention programs that will aim to advance these children and at the same time to empower their parents. Microcomputer-based interventions have the potential to meet the basic condition for empowerment programs, which was emphasized as enabling the individual to experience a sense of competence in a valued and challenging context.

Personal computers are rapidly becoming a part of our everyday life, entering work and home environments. The Special Education Technology Project of Tel-Aviv University in Israel, working jointly with various similar projects in the USA, has focused efforts on developing effective models for technology integration in special education systems. Parents who wished their disabled children to benefit from the advantages of technology and to be prepared for the transition into a society using computers, both supported the schools' efforts to include computers in their curricula, and at the same time urged the university project to view them as active participants in the process, extending the desired impacts in time and place. I believe that the case studies and examples cited in this book often constitute the best illustration of these families' difficulties as well as their courage and tenacity when facing the dilemmas and challenges of their daily lives. The families described, whose identifying information was modified in order to protect their privacy, accurately reflect the observed family configurations and dynamics.

Research demonstrated that presenting a computer to a disabled child will not create a significant change in his or her functioning. Only through a theoretically sound technology-supported intervention may we expect to witness a meaningful impact on the child's development. The significant role that parents may fulfill, in developing the age-related skills of their disabled children through the application of computer-supported interventions, may be a function not only of appropriate training, but also of parental ability to add new, demanding roles to their already existing overload of duties.

Given this growing need for a focus on the family perspective within a model for effective integration of technology into special education, the importance of presenting research data on the proposed individualized, dynamic intervention model is strengthened. The proposed model is adapted to parental needs and resources, with special emphasis on parental roles and the empowering process. As such, the volume is intended for researchers and practitioners across a wide array of fields who are interested in family research and parent empowering interventions, and for those involved in technology integration for youth in special education frameworks.

The book is divided into four major sections. The first section is concerned with providing an overview of the research related to effective integration of computers into the special education system. A cognitive approach for skill development, through various software programs such as drill-and-practice software, games and simulations, and word processing, is discussed. The second section is devoted to the application of the stress, resources, and coping model into families with disabled children. The suggested ecological approach highlighted the need for an empowerment model, adapted to individual needs. The third section deals with specific components of the proposed model, through surveys and case studies of families who participated in a series of studies, and with special emphasis on interactional aspects and parental roles. Finally, the last section provides a summary of the proposed interventional model, emphasizing future directions for research and experimentation.

The integration of computers into homes of disabled children has great potential to enhance the development of these children, and to empower their parents through introducing additional challenges into their already existing roles. My extensive research focusing on the family climate of these families in various ecological conditions highlighted the need for a multidimensional, dynamic approach to intervention planning. I hope that this book will help crystallize issues which may contribute to a better quality of life among these families.

Malka Margalit

# Acknowledgments

I wish to thank a number of people who helped bring this book to fruition. The research and case study descriptions presented in this book grew out of my work on the Special Education Technology Project at Tel Aviv University. I would like to express my many thanks to Yad-Avi-Hayishuv for their continuous help and support in this project. Special thanks go to Judith Rochberg and Hana Pinchas-Greenberg, whose devoted work as leaders of the parents' groups helped in exploring the advantages and difficulties related to the computer-supported intervention model. I also would like to acknowledge the superb editorial assistance provided by Dee B. Ankonina, who spent many hours reviewing the manuscript, and the enormous technical help provided by the research project staff. Finally, to the parents of disabled children who shared with us their moments of pride and sorrow, I relay my deepest appreciation for opening the door to our better understanding of their lives.

# Contents

## Section III The Entrance of Computers into Families

## Section IV Epilogue: Disabilities, Technology, and Families

# Section I

## Effective Technology Integration

# 1
# An Information Processing Model for Intervention

Change is an expression of contrast, a conceptual figure carved out of the ground of its unchanging counterpart (Mahoney, 1987). Any theory of human change will therefore need to address the complex dynamics of change and stabilization, taking into consideration the active role that persons play in sculpting their lives through experimentation, yet recognizing also the person's individual structure which may have a great impact on the person's ability or need for change. This paradigm of change appears all the more relevant for disabled individuals, who have often been characterized as passive in their interactions with the environment and whose capacity for change seems to be a function of the limitations of their handicaps.

Any intervention program rests on the supposition that human functioning is indeed flexible, and that the processes involved in human change are plastic (i.e., open to alteration). Clinical knowledge based on research and practice suggests that the success of preventative efforts and intervention programs may be greatly enhanced when the focus is placed on acquiring the skills for coping with current environmental demands and forthcoming transitions (Kendall, Lerner, & Craighead, 1984).

Efficacious treatment of childhood problems requires the additional understanding of developmental processes. How do these developing processes provide a changing range of opportunities in which experiences and/or interventions may alter individuals? How in this manner do individuals become part of the process of influencing their own change? Mahoney, in his comprehensive presentation at the 1987 American Psychological Association conference, emphasized the value of experience as a critical aspect of change. When children and adolescents do not explore and experiment in new ways of interacting with their internal and external environments, as often occurs with the handicapped, these youngsters are not likely to change.

## Processing deficiencies

A vast body of research (Kendall, 1987; Stone & Michals, 1986; Torgesen, 1982; Worden, 1986) has demonstrated that the source of many academic and behavior difficulties of mildly handicapped students lies in their deficient processing of environmental information. *Mildly handicapped* (Reynolds & Lakin, 1987) or *mildly disabled* students denotes students who are classified as educable mentally retarded, learning disabled, and mildly emotionally disabled (not psychotic or autistic).

Children and adolescents with disabilities have often been considered deficient in their information processing and problem solving abilities, hence they may be considered deficient in their ability to explore their environment and to learn about it. The basic deficits in the information processing of learning disabled and mildly mentally retarded students were attributed to four basic variables, in which mildly disabled students significantly differed from average students (Reschly, 1987):

1 Speed or efficiency in elementary information processing operations.
2 Knowledge base from previous learning.
3 Use of strategies in acquisition, memory, and problem solving.
4 Metacognitive operation.

The cognitive behavioral orientation most appropriately depicts disabled children's learning. This orientation emphasizes learning principles while also underscoring the importance of cognitive information processing variables (i.e., processing style, attributional patterns, and guiding schemata) in the learning process. Accepting the influential role of cognition in children's functioning, change introduction should focus on cognitive variables (Kendall, 1987).

In order to compensate for deficient cognitive processing among mildly disabled children and adolescents, a model of a cognitive human-machine interface should be developed, which would serve as a tool to increase the efficiency of human problem solving. The goals for intervention planning should focus attempts on increasing the speed and accuracy of task performance, expanding the amount of information available to the disabled student, and developing effective usages of cognitive and metacognitive strategies. Learning processes in the computerized environment can be structured, controlled, and accessible to experimentation and manipulations. The key consists of the effective application of computer technology, within an effective behavioral-cognitive oriented instructional model which supports the learner's efforts.

The integration of technology with procedures within the cognitive model necessitates research which should: (a) delineate the types of problem solving situations which consistently appear in this target group's environment and investigate these individuals' usual responses in similar situations, (b) evaluate what information these children and adolescents must know and how it can be used to solve these problems (Wood & Hollnagel, 1987), and (c) enable active experimentation to facilitate effective learning.

Section 1 aims to present the basic learning principles within the proposed information processing model in order to enhance effective usage of these computerized activities in the homes of disabled students, and to report results of research experimentation with preferred computer activities, emphasizing effective procedures.

## Basic learning principles

The study of human learning within the information processing model reveals a number of basic principles (Kendall, 1985; Mahoney, 1977):

1 The human organism responds primarily to cognitive representations and experiences in its environment, rather than to the environment and experiences per se.
2 Most human learning is cognitively mediated.
3 Thoughts, feelings, and behaviors are interrelated within any learning process.
4 Cognitive *contents*, *structures*, *processes*, and *products* are important in understanding and predicting behavior,

behavior difficulties, and interventions. Cognitive *contents* refers to the actual information (i.e., knowledge, events, self-statements) represented in memory. Cognitive *structures* can be identified as the manner in which the *contents* are represented in memory (i.e., schematic memory), thereby serving to filter and influence the processing of information input. Cognitive *processes* comprise the procedures by which the cognitive system operates (i.e., differentiations, identifications, distortions). Cognitive *products* constitute the results of the interactions of cognitive *contents*, *structures*, and *processes* (e.g., attributions).

5 Problem solving can be conceptualized as a goal-directed search among a variety of possible solutions within a specified problem space (Wertheimer, 1985).

Any intervention program for disabled students should be directed toward introducing change into these cognitive operations. Before initiating their learning activities, disabled students must develop clear goals and acquire a greater amount of facts and information, more effective procedures to monitor and reach these facts, and more efficient structures to manipulate and handle them.

## Training programs

A variety of interventions implementing the problem solving principle of the information processing model have been explored in recent research. Mayer (1987), for example, differentiated between the following types of skill training programs for enhancing efficient problem solving:

1 *Translation training* involves teaching the student how to transform the problem or each segment of information into an internal representation (e.g., understanding and memorizing the problem).

2 *Schema training* involves teaching students how to integrate the information into a coherent representation (e.g., knowledge of problem types, effective categorization of problems, diagrams, equations as representation).

3 *Strategy training* involves teaching the student how to devise and monitor solution plans, either in general- or domain-specific knowledge areas.

4 *Automaticity training* involves teaching students to effortlessly use the procedure and skill.

Disabled students often need these four types of skill training in order to achieve fluent performance in the academic and nonacademic tasks presented by school and home environments. Most intervention programs treat these training types as representative of different yet interrelated aspects of task performance, and their separate categorization here is provided only for academic purposes.

## The disabled as a novice problem solver analogy

An understanding of the source of disabled students' difficulties in schema development and strategy usage can be facilitated by the comparison between experts and novice problem solvers. Experts, approaching problems in ways that novices do not, possess complex problem representations or schemata that allow appropriate inferences to be made from problem statements. Experts' schemata consist of theoretical constructs that denote organized bodies of specific content-related knowledge (Beishuizen, 1988). The expert has more differentiated schemata, containing more connections to other related schemata (Halpern, 1987). In addition, the expert possesses clear, preprepared structures for representing large sets of organized information about concepts, thus facilitating inferences concerning both general concepts and specific structures which represent specific content areas (Anderson, 1985).

Individuals with disabilities, similarly to novice problem solvers, have global and less sophisticated schemata (Margalit, Weisel, Heiman, & Shulman, 1988), and usually have access predominantly to generalized problem solving strategies. In order to become an expert in any domain, a great deal of experience and practice is necessary, and instruction planning may play an important role during this practice in order to integrate general problem solving strategies with content-specific strategies.

## General and domain-specific strategies

Two types of strategic processing have been defined in the literature: general strategies and domain-specific strategies:

1. General strategic skills or general problem solving can be defined as learning general procedures that can be adapted to solving problems in different domain areas. Instruction in general strategies aims to enable the student to identify and classify problems, and to restructure, translate, and transfer knowledge and skills to new situations (Pfeiffer, Feinberg & Gelber, 1987).
2. Domain-specific knowledge and strategies can be defined as the *declarative*, *procedural*, or *conditional* knowledge one possesses relative to a particular field of study. *Declarative* knowledge refers to factual information (knowing what), whereas *procedural* knowledge consists of the compilation of *declarative* knowledge into functional units (knowing how). *Conditional* knowledge entails the understanding of when and where to access certain facts or employ particular procedures.

General problem solving training activities aim to train individuals who have difficulties in general cognitive and metacognitive skills and executive processing, as related to effective problem solving (i.e., selective attention, identification of problems and rules, planning, and understanding others' perspectives of performance).

Research in cognitive psychology during the last two decades has produced two undisputed findings about academic and nonacademic performance (Alexander & Judy, 1988) with implications for strategic processing. First, pinpointing the value of general strategies, learners who monitor, regulate, and manipulate information, using their general strategies and cognitive processing during task performance, do better than those who do not engage in such strategic processing (Flavell, 1981). Second, emphasizing the value of the domain-specific knowledge and strategies, those who know more about a particular domain, understand and remember better than do those with only limited background knowledge (Glaser, 1984). While these two findings have been consistently supported in research, there appears to be little understanding of how these two forms of knowledge and strategies interact during learning.

It seems that a certain amount of domain knowledge is necessary for the efficient and effective utilization of general strategic knowledge (Newell, 1980). Before the learner can apply general strategic knowledge to a domain task, in a manner that will facilitate completion, the learner must possess enough knowledge relevant to that domain. Children benefited from instruction in a general knowledge activation strategy when they possessed a high level of knowledge in the content area to which that strategy was being applied (Hasselhorn & Korkel, 1986).

The ways in which knowledge and process interact can provide significant benefits for training, if they constitute the target of detailed investigation (Sternberg, 1985). A need now exists to focus on these interactions, since research done in isolation on the benefits of either content-domain or general strategic approaches to problem solving demonstrated that both the "knowing" and the "knowing how to know" affect the performance of tasks.

## The acquisition of metacognition

Metacognitive processing may be defined as students' knowledge concerning themselves as learners and the regulation of learning activity. Two major changes in the development of the child may possibly contribute to the acquisition of metacognition. One is comprised by the development of the sense of self as an active cognitive agent, and as a causal center of one's own cognitive activity. The development of such an internal locus of control can promote the monitoring and the regulation of the child's own cognitive enterprises. A second kind of change that facilitates metacognitive development consists of an increase in planning abilities. An individual who represents and interrelates past, present, and future actions and events should be in a good position to acquire metacognitive knowledge. Such an individual can notice and store covariant person, task, and strategy factors. The mental age of the trained child is an important condition to be considered in the acquisition of metacognitive abilities. Adolescence may be viewed as the most advantageous developmental stage for focusing efforts on metacognitive training, as youth at this age are typified by growing self-realization and planning capacities.

The person who can look ahead also stands in a position to scan upcoming information or impending problems, and can plan in advance how processing resources should be allocated. Thus, an individual who can create conscious and explicit representations of the past, present, and future should be more appropriately equipped to make a better adjustment to his/her changing environment (Flavell, 1987). Another important factor emphasized by Flavell in his studies consisted of the finding that metacognition, like almost every other aspect of learning, development, and life in general, improves with practice. Through training in computerized activities, individuals with special needs may experience effective, content-free problem solving activities within a controlled (computer) environment, actively repeating their performance in order to reach automaticity.

## The optimal learning environment

The stable, controllable, and individualized nature of the computer contributes to its suitability for optimal learning among disabled children. Two additional characteristics of an optimal learning environment consist of the supportive adult (teachers/parents), and the externalization of internal structure. In several studies (Charles & Lester, 1984; Swing & Stoibel, 1988) it was found that the presence of positive, supportive, and effective teachers may be an important factor in the acquisition of knowledge. Another important social-contextual factor consists of the externalization of knowledge through thinking-aloud or dialogues. The teacher and the peer group have been found to solicit further elaborations or clarifications from learners or to provide them with feedback as to their performance (Smith & Good, 1984). This externalization of the cognitive processes, which has been found to have the effect of converting a highly private endeavor to a public one, has been shown to play an important role in optimal intervention.

## Conclusions

Children and adolescents with disabilities have been considered deficient in their abilities to explore environments and learn critical information. Their basic deficits in information processing were attributed to four main areas: (a) limited speed and accuracy in performance style; (b) a limited information base, and (c) limited cognitive and (d) metacognitive strategies. In order to compensate for these basic deficits, several types of computer-assisted skill training programs should be developed to enhance the following skills: translation, schemata, strategy, and automaticity skills.

The extent of the combination between two types of knowledge (i.e., contents specific to the problem, and general strategic knowledge) constitutes an essential component in learning. Different types of software can be used to train these two types of strategies, as can be seen on Figure 1.

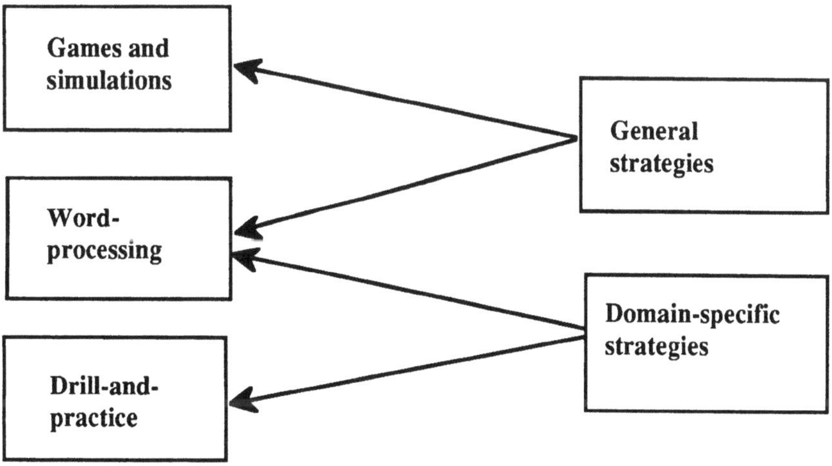


Figure 1.1. Home-computing and strategy training

In order to execute effective problem solving, an extensive body of domain knowledge must be accessible, and general strategies must be implemented. Metacognitive awareness of the relatedness between domain-specific and general strategic knowledge also comprises a crucial aspect of learning and retention.

Surveys of computer usages by mildly disabled students in different environments such as homes and schools (Cosden, Gerber, Semmel, Goldman, & Semmel, 1987; Goldman & Pellegrino, 1987) reported the three most frequent and preferred computer-integrated activities:

1 Drill-and-practice of basic skills
2 Games and simulations
3 Writing with word processors.

Computers have been used to increase knowledge in domain-specific areas via drill-and-practice programs and to facilitate the development of general strategic thinking through the use of games and simulations. The needs of disabled learners for help within these two approaches to learning will be presented as related to research results.

# 2

# Computer Games and Problem Solving

Playing computer games has been widely depicted as the most preferred computer activity reported by children with and without disabilities in both school and home environments (Carey & Gall, 1986; Swadener & Jarrett, 1986). The extracurricular use of computer games was an activity preferred by 61% of the boys and 54% of the girls in Swadener and Jarrett's (1986) study of middle-school children, and only 8% of that sample reported that they had never played computer games. These children viewed game activity as their preferred mode of computer usage not only in the present, but also in the future. Carey and Gall (1986) reported that for secondary school students, the use of the computer for entertainment and leisure activities predominated, with games as the preferred activity. They also found significant correlations between the types of computer usages at school and at home.

Computerized games and simulations are very attractive for children and adults. They challenge, stimulate curiosity, and contain fantasy (Malon, 1983). Children develop fluent game and simulation behavior through continuous playing, and they demonstrate successful strategies such as planning, predicting sequences, and improving outcome scores. With regard to special education students, two types of approaches can be applied toward game and simulation activity: (a) an emphasis on the game activities as a leisure activity, and (b) an instructional procedure to facilitate problem solving strategies.

## Leisure activity

Much research has recently been devoted to the leisure needs of disabled and nondisabled individuals. The industrialized Western society is moving quickly from being a work-centered to a leisure-centered society. This change means that work and work values will no longer be central in our value system, but will increasingly be replaced by leisure-oriented values. Westland (1987) suggested that as a result of the introduction of high technology in our communities, fewer workers will be needed for the production of more high-quality goods and services, resulting in sharply increased amounts of free time for individuals. This change will mean not only that those who are already involved in the production process will be needed for shorter periods of time, but also that growing numbers of people will be unable to become involved at all.

The expected increase of leisure time in the life of disabled individuals represents a specific area of difficulty. Even in our present societal conditions, learning disabled students have reported their inability to use their free time in an enjoyable and fulfilling manner. A survey of leisure activities among learning disabled students (Margalit, 1984) demonstrated that these students tended to be involved in passive, adult-dependent activities which were often evaluated as suitable for younger children. Parents reported that their disabled children often complained that when they were not participating in school or structured activities, they felt bored and awaited adult proposals of free-time activities. In order to develop meaningful and satisfying leisure activities, most mildly disabled students require an adult's instruction and guidance. Teachers and parents should plan and initiate age-appropriate activities that motivate and that do not foster dependence on adults.

Computer games and simulations may be viewed as an age-appropriate leisure activity which enables interactive performance and may even serve as a source of acceptable social interactions with peers, such as sharing and exchanging games or discussing successful strategies for solving adventure games. Although handicapped children may require parental support and encouragement in their initial game playing, such computer activities are often quite appealing to disabled learners, thereby facilitating the games' introduction into these children's leisure time. The integration of simulations and games, however, is valuable not only because they consist of a pleasurable means to spend unstructured hours, but also due to their potential contribution to problem solving abilities.

## Problem solving instruction

Many simulations and computer games demand effective processing of problem solving (i.e., concentration, planning, sequence prediction, and sensori-motor coordination). Observations have revealed that even children with learning difficulties, when provided with different levels of guidance and help, were able to develop fluent and automated play strategies. As games comprise a preferred activity, a critical question should be addressed: How may children's computer use at home be encouraged, not only as an active leisure activity, but also for promoting critical thinking abilities and effective problem solving? In order to study computer games and simulations as a means to facilitate cognitive processing, a model of schemata and executive processing will be discussed, and procedures for strategy instruction will be presented.

### Schema and structure

Information processing models assume that the successful comprehension of the environment involves the construction of an appropriate mental structure -- a schema -- that represents three major aspects: (a) the goals that can be satisfied by the execution of the operations contained in the schema, (b) the conditions under which the schema can be applied, and (c) knowledge of the structure and processes that are involved in the achievement of the schema's goals.

Within a dynamic process of selective attention and categorization, the individual imposes structure on incoming information from his/her internal and external environments. The individual then goes beyond the information given by the stimulus, filling in the gaps with information derived from memory, expectations, or inferences. The cognitive structures that mediate this organizational and inferential activity are known collectively as "schemata." Schemata refer to one's cognitive representations of past events, affecting present functioning.

Viewing individuals with learning disabilities as ineffective problem solvers has pinpointed research interest at their difficulties in developing appropriate schemata of the world. Confronted by complex, diverse, and fragmentary stimuli in the environment, they demonstrate difficulties in organizing the available information in an efficient and economical manner, in order to make use of it. In trying to solve a problem, the effective learner must employ thinking skills such as discrimination and classification; s/he may use inductive, deductive or syllogistic reasoning, and may need to order material in a linear or conditional form, using varying degrees of memory (Powell, 1987). Children with distorted schemata may require new experiences in carefully planned situations, along with guided interpretations and evaluations of the interactions, in order to facilitate both accurate schematic storage of the present events and necessary revisions of the already stored experience. An instructional procedure that aims at helping the disabled student to actively structure his or her environment and to impose effective schemata, may use computer games as a representative of a mini-world, with gradually increasing cognitive and performance demands.

## Executive processing

Many disabled individuals acquire the needed skills for controlled performance under controlled conditions, such as remedial settings and resource classes, yet continue to fail when faced with performing the task in their classroom or home. Executive processing seems to be critical for these individuals' adjustment. In order to maintain cognitive activity, which is subject to emotionally and motivationally determined variations, the human information processing system needs to structure not only schemata, but also executive decisions. The latter aim at the acquisition of information about ongoing cognitive activity and about the present state of one's cognitive endeavor, as well as about the transformation or maintenance of one's own cognitive activity and states.

Effortful cognitive processes, unlike automated processes, may vary in the efficiency of their organization and execution. Executive decisions are necessary in order to efficiently apply the growing repertoire of cognitive operations and to organize and execute effortful processes efficiently.

Executive decisions may be conceived as *condition-action* connections. *Conditions* correspond to internal representations of states during problem solving, such as the amount of solution effort invested, duration of search, type of problem, etc. *Actions* correspond to cognitive operations directed at the control and regulation of the solution process. Executive decisions may be considered as stored rules for the control and regulation of cognitive activities during the problem solving. For example:

> *If no progress is perceived, then resource investment must be increased for the solution search;*
> *If the goal cannot be reached, other strategies must be selected.*

Executive decisions are activated when certain states during the problem solving match up with stored knowledge (e.g., duration of efforts, length of search, type of plans, etc.). Knowledge about the connections between conditions and the manner in which actions perform, control, and regulate is assumed to be essential. In order to control or monitor cognitive activities, four types of executive processes are activated:

1 *Classification*: Provides an answer to the question "What am I doing here?" Identifies the type of problem.
2 *Checking*: Provides the answer to the question "How shall I do this?" Identifies how activities are organized, planned, memorized, progressed, and checked.
3 *Evaluation*: Provides information about the quality of the cognitive activities. Involves a criteria to be applied as the basis of judgment.
4 *Prediction*: Provides information about the alternative options for problem solving: the possible sequence of steps for solution and the potential outcomes. This type is especially needed in risky situations, in order to avoid extreme "costs." Refers to questions such as "How many letters can I remember?", "How well can I do this task?" etc.

These four hypothetical processes for controlling cognitive activities are not independent of one another. Evaluation requires checking, checking requires classification, and prediction requires checking. During the play with computer games, the individual may experience these four executive processes within the structured environment of the game situation. The instruction of problem solving should develop the player's insight into his or her goals and processing.

Executive regulation refers to decisions about organization, effort, amount, course, and direction of one's own cognitive activity. Regulation may be the cause for modifications, or for maintenance and continuation of the activity. The activation of the executive processes demands regulation of:

1 *Capacity*: The amount of effort that the individual is willing to invest in order to accomplish a cognitive demand, and the allocation of information processing capacity for mental operations. During the play activity, the individual becomes more motivated to invest efforts, and may experience his/her increased capacities, whereas during the traditional learning process, frustrations and failure may decrease the investment of effort.

2 *Content*: What segment should get more attention.

3 *Intensity*: Frequency of attempts, trials, time segments, solution searches, and different perspectives.

4 *Speed*: Varying pace, such as decreasing speed in difficult and new tasks.

The understanding of executive decisions and different processes serve as the foundation for the development of strategic instructional procedures.

## Strategy instruction

Learning to solve problems can easily be compared with learning to ride a bicycle or playing basketball. It requires active participation by the student and much time and practice. Teachers cannot "give" students a "gift" of effective problem solving skills (Pfeiffer, Feinberg & Gelber, 1987). Rather, general problem solving can be taught if teachers provide not only facts but also active practice and feedback. The role of the teacher lies in arranging the learning environment in a way that optimizes the student's activity during the learning experience. Structured opportunities including developmentally appropriate experiences in self-control and self-instruction should be planned in order to increase the likelihood of the desired outcomes. These opportunities can be provided through computerized activities. Software that produces interactive opportunities for children and adolescents may facilitate the active skills learning.

The purpose of strategy instruction may be viewed as: to influence how the learner interacts with the learning situation (Palincsar, 1986). General strategies that can be the aim of strategy instruction include guessing and checking, identifying salient features of the problems, recognizing patterns in the environment, working a problem backwards, mapping opportunities and drawing a picture-map of the problem, reasoning logically, discussing related tasks, self-questioning, and rejecting inappropriate solutions. Current information processing models claim that with repeated practice, many of the intermediate problem solving steps of both thought and action become fluent processing. A major determinant in achieving that development consists of the appropriate amount of experience with the problem solving activity, and technology may serve as a structured and controlled environment for that deliberate and planned experimentation (O'Leary & Dubey, 1979).

Strategies can be described as goal-directed procedures that are planned or intentionally evoked prior to, during, or after the performance of a task. Strategies aid in the regulation, execution, and evaluation of the task (Alexander & Judy, 1988). General strategic processing and strategic knowledge may exist separately from any specific content domain, and may be successfully applicable across many specific domains. At the same time, the student must be aware of how well the selected strategy is working. Disabled children's deficient metacognitive processing (i.e., their deficient knowledge about themselves as learners and their regulation of learning activity) has been viewed as a central target of computer-supported interventions, incorporating games and simulations.

Strategy training such as self-instructional training procedures are: (a) geared toward the development of self-guidance through practice with self-directed commands, suggestions, and rewards, and (b) focused directly on cognitive deficits (Kendall, 1977). Such interventions provide a cognitive strategy for the solving of problems -- a strategy that is either unavailable or not used prior to the training. Self-instructional training with children and adolescents is geared for cognitive absences: Teach the child who is not thinking how to think (Kendall, 1987).

## Motivational and affective aspects

Useful techniques for teaching problem solving fall into two important areas: providing students with a relevant and sufficient amount of experience in solving problems, and motivating students to solve problems (Pfeiffer, Feinberg, & Gelber, 1987). In order to motivate problem solving, students should face a challenge involving some difficulty and then should have access to the tools which can help them solve the problem more easily. Problems that appear too easy are unrewarding, and overly difficult ones do not allow the student enough success to be motivated, so that students tend to give up. Students must believe that they can solve the problem with a reasonable amount of effort, and expending that effort should be rewarding.

Another important task rests in making the challenge relevant, using familiar concepts and skills that have meaning for the students. One crucial motivational technique consists of the use of positive reinforcement:

*Praise the student for his/her achievement;*
*Emphasize the fact that making mistakes constitutes part of the learning process;*
*Reward students' positive efforts;*
*Gently point out errors;*
*Provide encouragement for additional experiments.*

The use of the computer enables the program planner to use these principles to ensure motivation. It should be clearly realized that when students also evidence a helpless attribution style, good metacognitive skills may not be sufficient for effective problem solving. Such an interaction between attribution bias and metacognitive knowledge calls for a detailed investigation in order to develop effective intervention plans.

## Survey of game and simulation research

A number of authors have suggested that the computer constitutes a powerful tool for the development of thinking skills and problem solving abilities in learning handicapped youngsters (Maddux, 1984; Russell, 1986; Schiffman, Tobin, & Buchanan, 1982). Although much has been written about the virtues of using the LOGO program with handicapped populations, too little empirical data exists to-date for conclusive statements on the advantages and disadvantages of using LOGO with handicapped students. As Torgesen (1986) pointed out, all of the evidence thus far on the use of LOGO with mildly handicapped children is anecdotal. Thus, considering the currently little evidence for LOGO's usefulness in the development of problem solving skills in learning handicapped individuals, it will not be the subject of the present discussion.

Much of the simulation software that claims to promote problem solving skills (e.g., planning, sequencing, following directions) has only remotely addressed these skills (Russell, 1986) and may be more appropriately classified as entertainment. However, several studies (Margalit, 1987; Margalit, Weisel, & Shulman, 1987) demonstrated that mildly disabled students improved their strategic thinking, as assessed on paper-and-pencil tests, following a training period with computer games. The training instruction integrated teaching self-instruction and self-verbalization strategies, developing metacognitive awareness and performing the instruction in pairs, using peer-tutoring. Significant differences were also found between a group of learning disabled children whose training emphasized strategic problem solving and metacognitive awareness, and a control group who simply played with computer games without a problem solving emphasis.

The results of these studies demonstrated that computer games and simulations presented within the framework of problem solving instruction can facilitate the information processing of learning disabled children. These results were found to be stable for the duration of five additional weeks without further training. The computer games provided the mildly handicapped children with an opportunity to experience problem solving in a structured and highly motivating environment. However, only the combination of that experience together with the instructional procedure affected this result.

Research comparing the use of conventional methods with the use of simulations to promote problem solving revealed mixed results, emphasizing the value of suitable instruction based on the problem solving model. Several studies did not find the simulation programs more effective than noncomputerized methods (Ellis & Saborinie, 1986), whereas others (Woodward, Carnine & Gersten, 1988) indicated significant differences in the children's problem solving skills, demonstrating the effects of transfer and maintenance. These mixed results imply that a more effective way to teach problem solving consists not of comparing computerized and noncomputerized simulations, but rather of emphasizing the instructional aspects. Ellis and Saborinie (1986) suggested that the direct tutoring of problem solving, followed by opportunities to practice the skills through simulation applications, may increase the students' achievements.

Hasselbring (1988) surveyed the research data regarding the application of computer simulations to teach problem solving and decision making skills. He also concluded that although the research evidence is limited, it pointed out that simulations may produce improved problem solving only when prior information is provided and can be used as part of the simulations. If the individuals are not informed and taught that these concepts and strategies are relevant to the problem solving activity, they may fail to benefit from the instruction. As problem solving skills constitute complex sets of action sequences organized in a coherent way in order to reach an intentional aim or goal (Beishuizen, 1988), teaching methods must be utilized to bridge these separate pieces of information toward the predefined goal and to increase the probability that appropriate information will be used in order to improve decision making and problem solving through computer simulations.

## Conclusions

Computer games were identified as the most preferred computer activity by children. Games and simulations provide an opportunity for the disabled student to be involved in an independent, age-appropriate activity either as a leisure activity, or as a part of problem solving instruction. The natural environment for games and simulations may be viewed as the home. Planned reinforcement from the family members, through a sequence of planned procedures, has potential to facilitate the transfer of problem solving skills from what may appear to some parents as a purely recreational activity. This attempt to encourage and reinforce the game and simulation activity, both as a legitimate leisure activity and as a possible facilitation of problem solving processing (i.e., structuring schemata, developing executive regulations, and teaching strategies), calls for a careful consideration of the family environment in families of mildly disabled children.

Game playing and problem solving experience through simulations may enable disabled students to progress in their process of developing effective schemata for problem solving and may activate their executive processing within a highly motivating learning environment. Research comparing the use of computer games and simulations, and of conventional methods for problem solving training, revealed mixed results, emphasizing the critical role of instructional procedures.

The research results suggested that two main characteristics of an optimal learning environment -- the supportive adults (teachers or parents) and the externalization of internal structure (schemata) -- should be considered for adoption in effective procedures for strategy instruction through computer games and simulations at home. In an attempt to achieve transfer of the problem solving skills into different tasks, and to facilitate the generalization and maintenance of the new skills, the development of a model for parents' training in strategic instruction should be the focus of further research efforts.

# 3
# Drill-and-Practice Programs

Computer-based drill-and-practice is designed to provide immediate corrective instruction, and to reinforce previously learned information, thus developing fluency or automaticity in the skill. In order to advance knowledge within the mastery-learning paradigm that assumes that most students can learn most things to a specific level of competence in varying amounts of time (Ackerman, 1987), the nature of the computer makes it irrefutably the ideal means for providing endless practice in a needed curricular area, until reaching the desired level of fluent performance.

## Controlled and automatic processing

In order to understand the critical importance of automaticity for learning, a comparison between a novice and an expert task performance provides a good illustration. The idea of distinguishing between the way subjects typically perform a novel task (i.e., in a slow, error-prone, and effortful manner) and how they perform the task after lengthy training or practice (i.e., quickly, accurately, and with little effort) (Ackerman, 1987) appears clearly to anyone who reflects on the differences between his/her own novice and practiced behavior in such situations as learning to drive a car or to use a word processor. The changes that take place, both quantitatively (e.g., in terms of task accuracy, speed, and amount of cognitive fatigue over task trial), and qualitatively (especially from a phenomenological perspective of effort demanded by the task), characterize the essence of the learning process.

The use of automatic processing is implied in the operation of various types of skilled performance such as playing the piano, swimming, and encoding words during reading.

Automatic processes are characterized as rapid, effortless (from a standpoint of allocation of cognitive resources), and unitized (or proceduralized), as they may not be easily altered by the subject's conscious control, yet they may allow for parallel operation with other information processing components within and between tasks. These processes may be developed only through extensive practice under consistent conditions. Consistency generally refers to (a) invariant rules for information processing, (b) invariant components of processing, and/or (c) invariant sequences of information processing components that may be used by the individual to attain successful task performance (Ackerman, 1987).

Individuals with disabilities often fail to develop automaticity in their skill performance, due to their need for more detailed and uniform training activities in order to reach such a performance level. Disabled learners' limited opportunities for experiences, in addition to their greater need for longer training periods, result in a failure to achieve the level of overlearning that leads to performance automaticity. Computers appear to provide an ideally suited invariant setting for training disabled students in automaticity. As a structured and controlled mini-environment which enables many repetitions, the computer may be adapted to individual needs with planned increases in complexity, until the child not only learns the skill, but also reaches the level of automatic effortless performance.

Although automatic processing has a very important value for special populations, controlled processing is neither less critical nor less necessary when the task requirements are novel, or when new elements enter into a well-known situation. Individuals with special needs often fail to acquire the automatic processing level of their nondisabled peers, and even if their training has reached such an automated level, they may demonstrate inappropriate automatic behavior when careful consideration of their performance is needed. Controlled processing is characterized as slow, effortful, and amendable to quick alternations under the subject's conscious control. The integration of technology into these types of learning processes enables the therapist to present the individual with a controlled, structured, and easily changeable mini-environment, in which to experiment and develop sensitivity to the interplay between the needs of automatic and/or controlled processing.

## Performance, resources, and limitations

With regard to the automatic and controlled processing theory, the notion of the performance-resource function postulated by Norman and Bobrow (1975) added an important perspective, providing critical concepts for understanding the sources of performance differences among groups of individuals with special difficulties and needs. Norman and Bobrow proposed two concepts reflecting the individual's and task's characteristics, and relevant to task performance: (a) performance limitations based on the amount of cognitive or attentional resources that the individual can devote to a task, and (b) performance limitations imposed by the task complexity and its difficulty level. In the automatic and controlled processing domain, the above limitations may be linked, respectively, with resource dependence and task dependence.

Novel tasks are more difficult, requiring controlled processing that may be dependent on personal resources. For a novel task that has the consistent characteristics necessary for the development of automatic processing components, task performance will gradually change from the resource-dependent stages of controlled processing to the first stages of automatic processing. After sufficient experience with the task, as automatic processing components develop, performance becomes less personal-resource-dependent. This stage is characterized by stable performance, regardless of the amount of cognitive resources devoted to the task.

For individuals with special needs, automatic processing that is less demanding on their personal resources may significantly compensate for their deficient cognitive processing. Lorsbach and Worman (1989), in their differentiation between explicit and implicit memory, further emphasized the importance of automaticity for learning disabled children. The children studied evidenced pronounced difficulties in their explicit, consciously effortful memory, yet during task performance which demanded implicit automatic memory, no differences were found between disabled and nondisabled children. Several investigators have proposed that attention constitutes a skill (Hirst, 1986; Hirst, Spelke, Reaves, Caharck, & Neisser, 1980), and that many different kinds of attentional skills exist (Hirst & Kalmar, 1987). The important interplay of controlled and automatic activities should not be ignored, and further exploration and investigation is required in order to understand their use in the learning process of special needs children.

## Survey of drill-and-practice research

The use of drill-and-practice software for developing automaticity has been documented as the single largest use of microcomputers in special education. Surveys of software programs for special education students in different age groups reported that drill-and-practice software was most frequently used, and most often in mathematics (Becker, 1986; Cosden et al., 1987; Goin, 1988; Rieth, 1986; Russel, 1986).

Without entering into the critical arguments against the stimulus-response nature of the drill-and-practice that makes students passive recipients rather than active initiators of learning (Turkel & Podell, 1984), it is commonly accepted that drill-and-practice comprises an unavoidable part of the curriculum for special education children, if they are to attain fluency in basic academic skills (e.g., math facts and sight word recognition). Torgesen (1984) argued that disabled students demonstrate difficulties in math and reading because they may have failed to master basic skills. In order to reach fluency and automaticity in these basic skills, extensive practice is needed for which the microcomputer is ideally suited. The basic assumptions about effective drill-and-practice programs include (Streibel, 1986):

1 Previous instruction in the concept or skill has already taken place.
2 There exists a right/wrong answer dichotomy in the logic of the content.
3 The basic unit of instructional interaction consists of a question-answer-branch episode. Continuous learner responses in the form of correct answers are therefore expected.
4 The feedback by the program also serves as an immediate check on the student's responses: positive feedback for a correct answer; and corrective feedback when the answer is incorrect.

Niemiec and Walberg (1987) reported that the review of research surveys on the effectiveness of drill-and-practice applications pointed out that special education children advanced their achievements more than nondisabled children. However, these authors pointed out the few studies existing in this area, stressing the need for more evaluative studies for disabled children. Another major theoretical aspect that remains to be studied consists of the relevance of basic skill training, in order to reach automaticity through drill-and-practice software, and to achieve the mastery of higher order learning performance.

### Fluency in mathematics

Drill-and-practice in basic mathematics comprises the academic software most commonly used by special education children. Its use is based on the assumption that the training of these children, until they reach automaticity and generalized math fluency, will free their thinking processing to focus efforts on solving mathematics problems requiring higher comprehension levels. However, several studies that have examined the use of different types of math drill-and-practice software, have reported that these programs failed to develop generalized math fluency and did not demonstrate clear advantages when compared with non-computerized learning (Christiansen & Gerber, 1986; Goin, 1988; Goldman & Pellegrino, 1987; Hasselbring, Goin, & Bransford, 1987; McDermott & Watkins, 1983).

Findings from these studies have shown that the use of these software programs resulted in some decreases in response latencies. However, upon a closer examination of the research data, this decrease can be mainly attributed to the students' greater efficiency at counting, and not due to the development of automatic recall of facts from memory. The mildly handicapped students in these studies were permitted to use controlled processes (i.e., calculating correct answers by using a process such as finger counting) for solving most problems. Hasselbring, Goin, and Bransford (1987) concluded that when mildly handicapped students employ counting strategies to solve math facts, developmental shifts whereby students begin to retrieve answers from memory are not produced by such drill-and-practice activities. The researchers suggested that drill-and-practice may be more effective if used only after students reach the level of mastery when they can retrieve the math facts from memory.

Another fluency training approach, the combined effect of tutorials plus drills on the math achievement of learning handicapped children, was reported in several studies (Hasselbring, Goin, & Bransford, 1987; Trifiletti, Firth & Amstrong, 1984) and was found to be more effective than resource room instruction. These studies emphasized that the combination of recall training with drills serves as a powerful mechanism for developing fluency in learning handicapped children.

Chiang (1986) reported that drill-and-practice software can be effective for teaching multiplication facts. A clear gain in multiplication mastery was demonstrated by Chiang through using 4-minute computer training sessions over a period of 12 days. He also found that the students transferred the skills practiced on the computer to paper-and-pencil tasks.

In an attempt to identify the relations between students' individual differences and mathematical gains from computerized drill-and-practice training, Ram (1988) performed a cluster analysis on 190 mildly disabled students mainstreamed into five regular schools, who participated in drill-and-practice training in mathematics. She identified three groups of mildly handicapped students: (a) students who were characterized by introversion, dependence on others, and low cognitive ability, (b) students whose main difficulties were behavioral and who were characterized by hyperactivity, aggression, hostility, and distractibility, and (c) students whose difficulties were less pronounced, either in behavioral or cognitive realms. The third group's computer achievements were the highest and were different from the former two groups. Differences in behavior and attitude toward the computer were found between the first two groups, yet no significant intergroup differences were found regarding achievement levels. The attitudes toward computer work among the students with behavior difficulties were less favorable, but their attitudes were not found to be significantly related to achievements.

The results of these studies highlighted the importance of remedial mathematic models to guide the development of drill-and-practice software, demonstrating their critical role in fostering the acquisition of significant achievements.

However, the assumption that the automatic mastery of basic mathematical facts will facilitate the learning of higher order problems has yet to be demonstrated. Two more critical aspects for the effective usage of math drill-and-practice software need to be investigated: (a) the teacher's role in facilitating the mastery of math facts and the integration of math software within the math curriculum, and (b) the role of the children's individual learning style in facilitating effective learning.

## Fluency in reading

In contrast to math drill-and-practice research, fewer studies have been conducted on the reading fluency of mildly handicapped students. It is commonly accepted that fluent decoding skills are essential for good reading comprehension, and the primary difficulties of mildly handicapped children are considered to be at the level of the word, rather than at the text level of processing. Torgesen (1986) suggested that reading instruction for mildly handicapped students should concentrate on activities that will strengthen their decoding and word reading skills, and that the text level of processing cannot be reached without initial fluent and automated decoding of words.

Practice with programs that trained in decoding skills (Roth & Beck, 1984) has resulted in significantly increased decoding skills and sentence reading speed. It appears that specific, well-designed training via the computer (e.g., practice in recognizing and analyzing words) is effective in increasing the fluency of the phonological decoding skills among this group of students. However, currently these results are too narrow to enable valid conclusions on the remediating of reading comprehension (Hasselbring, 1988). More studies are needed to investigate this approach, and especially to demonstrate the expected relation between automatic and fluent decoding skills and an increase in reading comprehension.

## Fluency in spelling

The results of attempts to use drill-and-practice programs to advance correct spelling have been mixed. Several studies (Fitzgerald, Fick & Milich, 1986; Haynes, Kapinus, Malouf, & MacArthur, 1984; McDermott & Watkins, 1983) demonstrated the advantage of computer-assisted spelling training to acquire correct spelling of word-lists, while others found in their studies that the achievements from spelling training with the computer were not significantly different from traditional training methods.

Another aspect of criticism lies in the observation that the automatic spelling performance reached through the practice provided by drill-and-practice programs differs greatly from the actual skill needed during the performance of a fluent writing task without spelling mistakes. Students were trained by computerized drill-and-practice software to use short-term memory to retrieve the correct spelling of lists of words, whereas during the actual writing task the students were required to automatically retrieve the correct spelling of words through long-term memory processing. Hasselbring (1984) reported that the application of a training procedure emphasizing the usage of long-term memory retrieval reached a spelling accuracy of 90% for the trained students. The advantages of this method were further demonstrated when voice-based spelling training was also integrated (Hasselbring, 1988). Margalit, Rot, and Greenberg (1988) further emphasized the importance of long-term memory training. They reported that the combination of keyboard training with an emphasis on the processing of word structure at the level of long-term memory retrieval improved spelling performance.

## Conclusions

Drill-and-practice software programs were designed to reinforce previously learned information, and to develop automaticity in basic skills. In order to advance knowledge within the mastery-learning paradigm, it is assumed that automaticity training may compensate for the students' learning difficulties, enabling them to focus their limited attentional resources on attempts to master higher order learning performance, such as reading comprehension. The conclusions from the research survey on computer-based training of mathematics, reading, and spelling skills emphasized the importance of the instructional planning, conveying that computer-based practice should be instructionally sound and should resemble the performance of the target skill as closely as possible. For instance, computerized spelling instruction should require the student to use long-term memory in order to succeed in the task, and mathematics training should be careful to avoid reinforcing inflexible counting habits.

Hasselbring (1988) suggested that other important characteristics of effective computer-based instruction which are in need of intensive research should not be neglected. For example, he advised placing limitations on the size of the practice set for each training session, spacing practice over days rather than having the student practice the same total time in one or two sessions, and emphasizing speed as well as accuracy. The use of computerized drill-and-practice programs at home may provide the disabled students with the amount of training sessions needed in order to reach automaticity and fluent performance. However, the studies' mixed results call for a careful selection of appropriate software and for planned monitoring of the training procedures in order to facilitate the achievement of the desired skills. Only through maximal coordination between school and home performance, including teacher-parent collaborations, may the effects of the drill-and-practice interventions at school and home be combined to advance basic skill fluency among disabled students.

# 4
# Word Processing and Writing Skills

Within most educational settings, writing serves as the primary means by which students demonstrate their knowledge, and it constitutes a powerful tool for recording ideas and exploring thoughts. Writing is also used as a common means of personal communication, fulfilling informational demands and emotional needs. In addition, writing has increasingly become a critical occupational skill: Successful performance in many occupations requires the ability to write in a clear and understandable manner.

Learning to write may be described as a particularly complex process. The shift from conversation to composition involves a radical conversion: generating language in the absence of a conversational partner; learning to activate relevant memories without having memories triggered by what someone else says; developing units of text larger than what is generally included in one conversational turn; and cultivating the ability to view what is produced from the perspective of both the sender and the receiver (Graham & Harris, 1988d). McCutchen (1988) identified various complex and demanding tasks in the writing process, involving many simultaneous subgoals and many interacting subprocesses, all of which vie for the attention of the writer whose cognitive resources are rather limited. Cognitive difficulties such as evident in learning disabled students may hamper the development of competent writing performance.

## Writing performance

Exceptional students typically exhibit poor writing performance, having difficulties not only in written expression, but also in handwriting and spelling. In addition, disabled students have considerable difficulties in executing and monitoring many of the cognitive processes central to effective writing, such as generating, framing, and planning texts. However, it is not surprising that the mechanical aspects of writing, such as spelling and handwriting, often receive the most attention in remedial settings, whereas the youngsters' ineffective writing strategies are neglected.

## Content generation

Handicapped students often produce written products that are inordinately brief (Deno, Marston, & Mirkin, 1982; Nodine, Barenbaum, & Newcomer, 1985). Their short written works seem to reflect not the students' limited knowledge, but rather their difficulty in accessing the knowledge they do have, and in expressing their ideas. These disabled students can be described as having content generation problems, where they have failed in employing self-directory strategies for a memory search. MacArthur and Graham (1987) also found that disabled students may possess more knowledge than is reflected in their written products. When these students were encouraged and asked to write more, or even when they were able to dictate their ideas instead of writing them, their works were found to be three to four times longer than those papers written via handwriting or word processing. Exceptional students' difficulties in retrieving ideas were also evidenced by their failure to produce multiple statements about familiar subjects (Thomas, Englert & Gregg, 1987). Training students in brainstorming or idea generation techniques may assist them in their efforts to develop their compositions' contents. However, students, especially disabled learners, also require a structured context in which to frame their ideas.

## Structured knowledge

In order to meet the demands inherent in a particular writing task, good writers commonly develop an ongoing frame for their text by using their knowledge of genre patterns or other discourse schemata to decide what information to include in their writing and to regulate the sequence of various ideas.

Disabled students often lack this frame of work. As a result of their lack of structured knowledge regarding how to go about the writing process, each new writing task seems to be a completely new task, arousing a pattern of anxiety and feelings of helplessness. For the disabled child, writing can be considered a dead-end process, rather than a gradual development of communication abilities (Morocco, 1987).

Exceptional students often lack the cognitive strategies that more experienced writers use for managing these basic experiences. Although these students appear to be somewhat successful in using a knowledge of genre patterns to develop and frame text, as evidenced by their ability to generate compositions that contain at least some elements common to the type of writing they are assigned (Graham & Harris, 1988a), their structural knowledge may be described as either incomplete or not accessed. Their compositions frequently fail to include critical elements such as the ending to a story, or the conclusion to an essay. Furthermore, a considerable amount of irrelevant or nonfunctional information is often generated. Thus the students' ability to use genre-specific knowledge to retrieve and organize relevant information appears to be limited. Thomas, Englert, and Gregg (1987) reported that learning disabled students often approached writing by converting the assigned writing task into a question-answering task in an associative sequence. A student using a planning strategy of this nature will direct little attention to the needs of the reader, the constraints imposed by the topic, and the whole-text organization of their written composition.

The lack of facility with the basic mental processes needed in writing is usually coupled with anxiety after several years of failure (Morocco & Neuman, 1986). The frustrated writers attempt to avoid writing in general and often approach writing tasks in an impulsive manner, trying to complete assignments by writing the minimal amount necessary. Consequently, they spend insufficient time with written communication in order to acquire greater proficiency.

## The advantages of word processing

Word processing has four key features that may affect the quality of writing performance among exceptional students (MacArthur & Shneiderman, 1986):

1 The ability to produce neat work.
2 The possibility to make frequent editions or revisions without tedious recopying, enabling the student to concentrate on content and to postpone his/her struggle with organization, style, and mechanics to a later time.
3 The relative ease of typing in comparison to writing by hand for many students with motor coordination difficulties.
4 Specific capabilities provided through programs related to the word processor, such as spelling checkers, talking word processors, and programs with the aim of generating ideas at the pre-writing phase.

Effective programs for improving the writing performance of mildly handicapped students are needed if they are to successfully cope with writing demands and with minimal competency testing requirements in educational systems (Graham & Harris, 1988c).

## The value of writing at home

The development of writing fluency is dependent on the opportunity to write, requiring, in addition to proper motivation, well-designed and carefully sequenced instruction and guidance as well as sufficient time for practice in the development of relevant skills and strategies. In their instructional recommendations for developing writing programs for exceptional children, Graham and Harris (1988d) emphasized the importance of adequate time in order to achieve writing mastery. Students can develop this competency only through writing experience. Yet in the study of writing instruction, learning disabled students were found to spend less than 10 minutes per day actually composing. The failure of school systems to allocate sufficient time for writing, as a result of limited computer availability in most educational settings, has a profound impact on exceptional children's writing development and composing achievements.

Bos (1988) proposed another critical component in successful composing: the creation of an environment that provides time to think, reflect, and write. This stands in obvious contrast with typical practice in many regular and special education classrooms, where students are expected to complete a written product within a short period of 30 to 40 minutes. Bos suggested that students should be encouraged to write for longer units of time, and even to continue working on the same piece of writing for more than one session. The opportunity to continue a writing task at home may be an appropriate solution to the need for longer computer access time periods allocated to writing tasks, enabling the student to think and reflect without time constraints.

Graves (1983) pinpointed an additional important aspect in the creation of an optimal writing atmosphere: an emphasis on the student's sense of independence and on limited teacher direction. This recommendation seems contradictory to exceptional children's greater need for extensive writing instruction; it appears impossible to appropriately integrate dependent, directed work with independent student work during the short time periods that computers are available to these students for writing tasks. However, home-school coordination can be planned where the classroom will provide intensive instruction and individualized guidance, and the student's work during the longer periods of computer time at home will be characterized by independence from teacher supervision and freedom from distracting factors such as peers, noise, and time pressures. An instructional approach that may integrate writing performance along a school-home continuum may serve as an appropriate solution to the need for allocating longer, more frequent writing opportunities which offer an interplay between dependent and independent student functioning. Such an approach calls for careful consideration of parental roles in supporting the instructed writing strategies while simultaneously allowing, and even encouraging, independent performance. In order to review the aforementioned approach, the results of previous studies investigating exceptional students' word processing instruction will be discussed.

Coe's (1988) observations revealed that young children at home write by choice, and this self-initiated writing may differ from assigned writing tasks in school settings. Young writers may write for a variety of purposes, and teachers often overlook such products, or deny their importance as "real" writing. Children learn to write by attempting a wide range of functions and genres, and not exclusively by writing stories. Young children attempt a wide range of functions and kinds of writing in their homes, and their parents' responsiveness may affect their writing.

Two important aspects of a print-rich supportive home environment have been also identified: (a) the presence of a role model who conveys the value of regular writing as part of everyday transactions and (b) the availability of an audience that evidences interest and responds to the child's productions. Research comparing home and school cultures as a social context for learning about writing have highlighted the value of a supportive environment for writing.

## Survey of handwriting and word processing research

Research on the use of word processors with exceptional students has been rather limited to-date. However, the results of several studies (Fais, 1987; Kerchner & Kistinger, 1984; MacArthur, 1988b; Morocco & Neuman, 1986; Sitko, 1988; Sitko & Crealock, 1986) have revealed that the use of word processing with writing instruction has resulted in increases in the quality and quantity of exceptional students' written work and positive attitudes toward writing. The concept of the computer as a "prosthetic device" was suggested (Sitko, 1988), conceptualizing the word processor as a necessary rather than optional aid for mildly disabled students and as a consistent part of their life-long effort to achieve maximum writing performance rather than as a temporary support. Sitko found that word processing even served to improve the learning disabled students' writing more than the nondisabled's students' writing, and the significance of this finding was emphasized from a cost-effective point of view in educational planning.

Although the previous review of the research concluded that procedural writing instruction has high potential for teaching writing to mildly handicapped learners, the question of whether students write less successfully when the word processor is not used should also be examined. Vacc (1987), in a study of mildly mentally retarded adolescents, found that when word processor use for letter writing was compared to handwriting, the students spent significantly more time using the word processor and wrote longer letters, making substantially more revisions. However, the mean number of words written per unit of time spent working on writing a letter was significantly higher for subjects' handwritten letters. While judges' holistic evaluations of letter quality did not differ significantly between the two production modes, it should be remembered that the holistic scores assigned to all these letters tended to cluster near the lower end of the rating scale, and thus failed to differentiate between the two groups.

Morocco's research (1987) recommended the use of word processing, emphasizing that: (a) learning disabled students using word processing tended to write longer compositions, since they did not have to recopy their written work, and (b) the interactive feature in word processing writing enables the teacher to add comments without interfering with the students' feelings of privacy, as the word processor was perceived as a more public instrument than the students' pages.

Graham and Harris (1988d) also reported improvement in the writing performance of exceptional students via training on the word processor. Their written essays were considered to be qualitatively and quantitatively better after training, and were found to generally include all the components considered central to the essay. Essays were usually longer and the text was more coherently ordered. In addition to the improveming their essay writing, the students participating in the study demonstrated more self-confidence in their ability to write and revise a good essay.

The conclusions of most studies accentuated two major conclusions relating to word processing:

1 The simple provision of a word processor without modifying instructional methods will not improve handicapped students' writing. The value of word processing for handicapped students depends on how effectively the instructional program takes advantage of the computer's capabilities for supporting students during the writing process, as well as on the students' specific cognitive processing dysfunctions.
2 Individual differences between the disabled students, expressed in their writing style and in the consistency of their improvements, constitutes the source of evaluation difficulties, highlighting the importance of the structured case study methodology for these

> studies. The critical question seemed to be not "Is using a word processor advantageous for the disabled student?" but rather "What are the optimal writing conditions for different disabled students?"

## The role of strategy training in writing instruction

Ellis and Sabornie (1986) compared students' writing under three conditions: (a) handwriting, (b) word processor, and (c) word processor plus idea processor (outlining program). The results of the study showed that prior to the strategy training there were no differences between handwriting and word processor conditions. However, the word processor plus the idea processor produced more positive results. Following strategy training, the students' writing improved under all three conditions, with the word processor plus the idea processor again showing the best results. Ellis and Sabornie concluded that generic strategy training (e.g., outlining) was better than no training; however, specific strategy training was especially superior when paired with the computer.

The model proposed by Morocco (1987) also portrayed specific linkages between procedural instruction and many of the writing outcomes that are critical for learning disabled students: productivity (number of words), a sense of ownership regarding the writing, and metacognitive awareness. Her students were aware of their cognitive processing during writing, expressed pride and enjoyment from the writing performance, and wrote longer compositions.

Fais (1987) in his studies further differentiated between holistic and specific measures of writing evaluation. He reported on the Forman School Computer-Aided Writing Project, designed to validate the effects of using computers to enhance the writing skills of learning disabled students. Twenty-seven students who participated in the study produced informal writing samples and were tested on their abilities to (a) judge the relevance of specifics to a given topic; (b) categorize specifics and topics into coherent groupings/ outlines; (c) order specifics in a logical paragraph sequence; and (d) proofread a paragraph not only for grammatical, punctuation, and spelling errors, but also for mistakes in organization and clarity. In addition, the students were administered pre- and post-assessment procedures consisting of four sections of the Test of Adolescent Language (TOAL), which examined their grammatical abilities in the areas of reading, listening, speaking, and writing.

During the experiment, the students spent one day each week for nine months working on the word processor within a structured writing instruction program that emphasized idea generation and outline formulation. The results of the study demonstrated that all the improvements in pre-post assessments occurred in the paragraph-sized tasks: organizing specifics into paragraph form, proofreading, spelling, written grammar, and spoken grammar. Students showed a much greater tendency to make appropriate corrections on the proofing task. Teachers reported that the students were using a more sophisticated vocabulary and sentence structure, generating much greater quantities of written material. However, students' performance on tasks isolated from the holistic paragraph context (e.g., crossing out unrelated specifics in a list, categorizing/outlining items in a list) and on the receptive tests of reading grammar and listening grammar showed no improvement. The improvement in active expressive writing tasks seemed to point to a positive experience in the interaction with the word processors. The fact that the passive and task-specific post-tests did not demonstrate improvement may indicate that these isolated tasks are not necessarily critical to the writing process, suggesting that researchers should be alerted to the difficulty of designing valid and reliable evaluative assessments.

The results of Kurth's (1988) study indicate that even very young children can benefit from careful word processing instruction in composition writing. These findings corroborated previous research results which emphasized that only a combination of high quality writing instruction along with the word processing can lead to improved writing. It was again found that working with word processing alone will not automatically increase the quality and the quantity of exceptional students' compositions writing. The most important ingredients in any composition program seem to be a sequenced, individualized instructional program and a teacher who is knowledgeable about composing processes.

## Procedural writing instruction

Procedural instruction may be considered critical throughout the writing cycle, because it provides children with the knowledge of how to plan, compose, review, edit, and even print their writing. The model begins with the point at which the student confronts a writing task. Writing always consists of an act of inquiry, and it can be viewed as a call to think. Students respond differently to that call, depending on their ability to bring planning, composing, and reviewing procedures to their writing process. Sitko (1988) identified three major elements in the writing outcome: Cognitive expectancy, production support (i.e., typing abilities and word processing skills), and composition support, including vocabulary (topic) and structure (genre).

The survey of the writing research has focused attention on the following processes applied in procedural writing:

1 Prewriting activities
2 Composing activities
3 Editing and revising

## Prewriting activities

The structured instruction of writing pinpointed attention at the importance of prewriting activities. Several skills are necessary to enable efficient writing performance, such as machine skills, planning skills, strategy training, and training in automatic vs. controlled processing.

### Machine skills

Most studies on writing composition (Dalton, Morocco & Neale, 1988; Sitko, 1988) have reported that students require sufficient keyboard skills and knowledge of basic word processing functions (i.e., cursor movement, capitalization, indent, delete) before beginning real composing activities; otherwise their work will be interrupted. Slow typing and confusion about saving procedures, loading files, and formatting texts may need special attention and training. Two training approaches have been described: (a) teaching these skills separately prior to the writing instruction, and (b) devoting only a very short period of time to introducing these skills before initiating writing instruction, and then instructing the keyboard and word processing skills only when the need arises.

Dalton, Morocco, and Neale (1988) reported that the teachers in their three research sites devoted special attention to teaching such basic word processing features as cursor movement, delete, insert, and file management (e.g., save, retrieve, and print). However, the amount of time and type of instruction varied widely among the teachers. Several teachers taught a sequence of group lessons, where they demonstrated the use of a specific word processing function and then prompted the students as they practiced the procedure on their own computers. Other teachers helped students with word processing skills as the need arose.

Machine skills seemed to remain a major preoccupation for most students, interfering with the teachers' attempts to focus primarily on writing issues after a brief initial period of keyboard skill instruction. Although the majority of the students typed in a relatively easy and quick manner after several months of work, it became evident that those students who received no direct machine instruction appeared fairly competent on the keyboard during the first few months, when writing assignments were relatively short, but demonstrated their weak machine skills during the latter part of the year when they began to write more extended pieces on the computer.

Based on these observations, Dalton, Morocco, and Neale (1988) recommended an approach to teaching machine skills that includes several guidelines and a model for balancing attention to writing and word processing:

1 Teach keyboarding for a minimum of three weeks, with short frequent practice sessions, prior to any teaching of word processing skills.
2 Devote four to six weeks to teaching carefully monitored basic word processing skills. These skills should include typing text and using basic file management functions.
3 Introduce advanced revising and editing skills (i.e., center, block move, find and replace, block erase and

copy) only as they are required to accomplish specific writing objectives.

MacArthur and Graham (1987) found that proficiency in typing was highly correlated with length, quality, and structure of the composition. The explanations offered by information-processing theory for the observed decline in writing abilities when children learn new word processing skills clarify the importance of careful consideration regarding machine skills training. The introduction of a new word processing task places additional demands on writers, requiring that they attend to both the writing task and the word processing task. This may overload the exceptional students' limited processing capacities, resulting in a temporary decline in writing performance while attention is concentrated on learning the new machine skills. As writers move from an effortful stage of skill acquisition to a more fluent stage of independent skill application, they are able to gradually increase the attention given to the writing skill. Automatic usage of the machine skills may thus enable exceptional students to devote their rather limited cognitive resources to writing.

## Planning

Prewriting activities address writers' needs to plan their writing. Morocco and Neuman (1986) suggested several guidelines for the student in the prewriting phase:

1 Defining and focusing on a topic.
2 Anticipating audience needs.
3 Generating ideas.
4 Organizing information.

Craig (1987) suggested that prewriting procedures should include the students' and teachers' brainstorming of topics for writing. He emphasized that prewriting constitutes a different process for different people; some start by typing ideas, others may outline a format, and still others may use mapping. Mapping entails a visual/hierarchical structure to show relations between ideas. Some students found the use of grids to generate specific components for narratives very helpful.

The structure of stories (story grammar) can be reduced to two major components: setting and episode (Graham & Harris, 1988b). The setting typically incorporates three elements: introduction of the main character, description of the locale, and information about the time frame of the story. Episodes introduce and resolve the plot of the story and usually include five elements: starter event (occurrence of a precipitating event), goal (the main character's reaction to the precipitating event and formulation of a goal), action (a planned effort to achieve the goal), ending (the results of the action), and reaction (emphatic statement or final response of a story character to the consequences of the action).

The conclusions from the several studies surveyed guided the procedural instruction of prewriting through presenting disabled students with the following six main questions regarding character attributes, time, location, and plot activity:

*Who is the main character?*
*When does the story take place?*
*Where does the story "happen"?*
*What does the main character do, and what happens?*
*How does the story end?*
*How does the main character feel?*

The disabled student should keep the 6-question structure in mind at all times, utilizing the questions as organizing milestones for thought and planning. The importance of maintaining a fixed, structured plan in consciousness -- even rigidly -- for all of the student's writing activities should be emphasized. At the same time, in using the 6-question structure, the student should devote equal effort to include new, innovative, creative additions and modifications to the story, so that each composition can be considered uniquely original. This interplay between formal structure and flexible modification comprises the essence of good planning for a writing composition.

## Strategy training

Graham and Harris (1988b) reported on the efficacy of strategic instruction in facilitating the generation, framing, and planning of text. Students were taught a series of self-directed prompts that required them to: (a) consider their audience and reasons for writing, (b) develop a plan for what they intended to say using knowledge of discourse schemata or frames to generate and organize writing notes, (c) evaluate possible content generation, and (d) plan during the actual act of writing. The self-instructional strategy training procedure was applied, using self-statements designed to support and regulate the smooth execution of the strategies, and providing the rationale for their use.

Graham and Harris (1988a), in order to further structure the strategy training in writing, provided their students with the following 3-step writing strategy:

1 Think: Who will read this and why am I writing this?
2 Plan what to say using *TREE*:
T.....note *Topic* sentence,
R.....note *Reasons*,
E.....*Examine* reasons,
E.....note *Ending*.
3 Write and say more.

This strategy requires writers to consider their purpose, their reasons for writing the composition, and their audience. Writers must evaluate writing content by considering the potential reader, generate notes that correspond to the basic components of a good essay, and continue the generation of content and planning during the actual writing.

Cognitive-behavioral theorists have proposed that effective strategy training involves three major components: strategies, knowledge about the use and the significance of those strategies (meta-strategy information), and self-regulation of strategic performance (Brown & Campione, 1986; Brown, Campione & Day, 1981; Pressley & Levin, 1986). Multi-component strategy training interventions based on this theoretical view have proven efficacious in improving performance, and frequently in obtaining generalization and maintenance among young children and disabled students. Self-regulation procedures have also been effective in increasing children's self-efficacy (Bandura & Schunk, 1981). This approach has been successful in improving written language skills among learning disabled students (Case & Harris, 1988; Graham, Harris & Sawyer, 1987; Harris & Graham, 1985).

Elliott-Faust and Pressley (1986) demonstrated that multi-component training, including a complete and effective strategy embedded in a self-instruction domain-specific routine, combined with self-monitoring of strategy use and effectiveness, was superior to simply teaching children the task strategy. Graham and Harris (1988b) found that self-instructional strategy training produced meaningful and lasting effects on subjects' composition skills as well as a significantly heightened sense of self-efficacy.

### Automaticity vs. controlled performance

Another skill training aspect that should be considered at this prewriting stage is related to automatic versus controlled processing. Automated procedures have two salient characteristics: (a) They demand fewer resources to operate; and (b) they become highly routinized and thus difficult to penetrate or break apart into components (Anderson, 1983). The skilled writer (McCutchen, 1988) seems to possess fluent language generation procedures, but these procedures appear to be far from being automatic. Automaticity may lead to encapsulated language generation procedures, placing the procedures beyond the reach of processes for metacognitive control over the subprocesses involved in writing.

Automaticity in machine skills can be considered desirable, freeing exceptional students to dedicate their efforts to the planning process. However, in idea generation procedures, the educational aim may be described as fostering sufficient fluency while at the same time keeping those procedures open to metacognitive processes that must disrupt them. A balance is needed between fostering fluency and encouraging metacognitive awareness of the writing process.

## Composing activities

The brevity of the description of the actual composing stage reflects the lengthy, comprehensive work devoted during the prewriting stage. Composing includes translating thoughts and speech into text, and expanding the initial text, key words, prewritten ideas, and writing plans (Craig, 1987; Morocco &

Neuman, 1986; Sitko, 1988). During the composing stage, efforts are mainly focused on the content and clarity, and writers are encouraged to write as fluently as possible, ignoring structural considerations, and concentrating all efforts onto expressing written ideas. Increased emphasis on the prewriting stage may help to enable fluent processing during this composing stage.

## Editing and revising the composition

The computer constitutes a flexible writing tool that eases the physical burden of revising and editing by eliminating the need for tedious recopying. However, it is important to recognize that revising in itself comprises an elaborate cognitive process that requires students to review their work, diagnose problems, and rewrite more effectively. The simple provision of editing possibilities has not been found to affect the writing performance of disabled students. No differences were found between word processing and handwriting conditions in the revisions performed by learning disabled students (MacArthur, 1988a), with regard to the number of revisions and their impact on the quality of the work. However, students' writing did improve when through careful and planned writing instruction they learned specific strategies for revising their work. The results of the study lead MacArthur (1988a) to suggest the following strategic steps in order to teach disabled students to perform meaningful revisions:

1. *Read your essay.*
2. *Find a sentence that expresses what you believe: Is it clear?*
3. *Add two reasons why you believe it.*
4. *Use the SCAN strategy for each sentence:*
   *S - Does it make Sense?*
   *C - Is it Connected to my belief?*
   *A - Can I Add more?*
   *N - Note errors.*
5. *Make changes on the computer.*
6. *Reread the essay and make final changes.*

Morocco and Neuman (1986) suggested on the basis of their studies that editing instruction should also involve the application of writing conventions for spelling and mechanics.

## Individual differences and specific facilities

Disabled students have revealed varied writing profiles and heterogeneous difficulties, and therefore respond differently to writing procedures and uses of word processing. For students with motor coordination problems, and those whose major problem consists of illegible handwriting, typing can be a great advantage in comparison with handwriting.

Spelling checkers may help students with spelling difficulties. The student who is freed from worrying about the correct spelling of words may devote more efforts toward composing. However, the usage of this additional program poses several procedural possibilities, and research is needed to investigate the optimal procedures for adopting the spelling check options. The advantages and disadvantages of the automatic spelling checker when used during the writing process versus during checking at the final editing stage should be studied.

Highly creative but distractible students may thrive on composing directly onto the word processor, provided they have a structure or a framework to focus their attempts. An idea processor combined with the word processor may assist in schema development. Research (Ellis & Sabornie, 1986) has demonstrated the advantageous usage of this combination with and without procedural instruction of writing.

Students with reading difficulties may use word processors with synthesized speech output to assist their revision work. Speech output permits inexperienced or poor writers to use their relatively stronger auditory language skills to monitor their writing. Rosegrant (1986) studied the use of a talking word processor and found that the students who used it, in comparison to students who used the regular word processor, spent more time in writing, made more revisions, and produced texts that were longer and higher in quality. MacArthur (1988b) viewed the talking word processor as a means to support a holistic approach to writing instruction that focused on meaningful communication rather than on isolated skills instruction. Kurth (1988) also found that the use of word processing with voice synthesis may be most suitable for beginning writers or for low ability readers as they begin to write. However, he found that for expert readers it is not as useful as expected. These students very soon found that the use of the voice synthesis takes more time than their own reading of their compositions, and they stopped using the voice output. Yet, the slow readers continued using it as a support for their work.

For some students, the use of word processing serves as a source of further anxiety. Highly anxious students may produce even less original text on the computer, because of the visibility of whatever they write and the ease with which they can erase. These students may need to develop confidence off the machine before using this more public writing tool.

## Conclusions

Children need several kinds of knowledge in order to carry out the writing process: substantive knowledge (ideas, content, information); procedural knowledge (ways to manage and carry out planning, organizing, composing, revising, editing); and skills (rules for correct mechanisms, and machine skills). The writing process can be viewed as a cycle, where each increment in productivity, sense of ownership, and metacognitive awareness provides students with a greater ability to call on planning procedures with each new writing task.

Disabled students often revealed difficulties in their writing performance, and the structural writing instruction using word processing may help them in fostering their writing skills. Exceptional students may have knowledge and experience to draw on, but often they have difficulty accessing, organizing, and transcribing it. For these students, acquiring procedural knowledge through teaching the various stages of prewriting activities such as keyboard training, planning and strategic performance and post-writing stages of editing should be viewed as extremely important. The balance of substantive and direct instruction with procedural instruction appears critical to empowering these disabled writers. Research demonstrated the advantage of word processing for writing performance especially for the disabled students, but further emphasized the value of structured instruction. Individual differences and needs were also met by the special provisions of word processors, such as the spelling checker, the talking computer, and the idea generator.

Writing comprises a time-demanding activity, and the limited machine time available in school settings imposes special difficulties. Writing at home presents the opportunity for having more time and greater independence from interfering classroom stimuli. The advantages of using word processing in the home environment are dependent on defining a meaningful parental role for supporting the procedural writing, while enabling a sense of ownership and independence for the disabled writer. Home-school interrelations are needed to advance the children's writing, thereby fostering the continuation of the school writing performance at home. The research on the various aspects of the home environment in families of mildly disabled children, as related to support for the disabled students' writing and composing, has special importance.

# Section II

## Families: An Ecological Model

# 5

# Familial Stress and Resources

Computers can be used to develop the skills of mildly disabled children, expanding their rehabilitation opportunities. The usage of computers at home may be regarded as an answer to the increased needs of these children for longer training periods, providing them with almost unlimited computer time. However, the simple provision of home-computers to these children has not been found to affect their performance, similarly to findings in the school setting. Role definitions and involvement levels of significant adults in structuring the computerized learning environment appears to be an important factor in advancing child-computer interactions. The extent to which parents affect their children's computer-assisted activities may be related to a number of individual and family variables, such as the effects of the prolonged stress experienced by these parents, and the resources available to these families. Exploring variables present in the ecology of a handicapped child, with a focus on a stress, resources, and coping paradigm, will lead to a more comprehensive understanding of these families (Short-Degraff, 1987).

Families of mildly handicapped children often experience high levels of stress (Dyson & Fewell, 1986; Friedrich, Wilturner & Cohen, 1985). Researchers have attempted to identify two groups of factors related to stress: factors that contribute to increased feelings of stress, and factors that serve as buffering mechanisms which mediate the effects of stressful life events (Crnic, Friedrich & Greenberg, 1983; McCubbin, 1979). Section 2 aims to discuss the concept of family ecology and resources for coping with stress, which provides a powerful explanatory model for the adaptation of families with handicapped children, directing intervention programs in general, and computer-assisted programs in particular. The study of these family members' resources, and of their needs for developing new roles and for adapting their coping skills to new and increased demands, may serve as guideposts for the development of comprehensive intervention planning. We now appear to be standing at a crossroads, where innovative and responsive models for computer-assisted interventions in the family have the capability to accommodate the growing knowledge of family systems and of individual aspects within families of mildly disabled children.

## Stress

Stressors have been defined by Antonovsky (1979) as demands: (a) made by the internal or external environments; (b) which tax or exceed the resources of the individual or the system, upsetting its homeostasis; and (c) which lack readily available automatic adaptive responses. Stress associated with the presence of a handicapped child is likely to be related to the family's cognitive appraisal of the stressful situation (Lazarus, Kanner, & Folkman, 1980) and to the family's available resources (Folkman, Schaefer & Lazarus, 1979). The following case study of a family with a disabled child exemplifies the stress and resources paradigm:

*Case study: The A. family*

*Mr. and Mrs. A. viewed themselves as successful people in their professional life and competent parents to their two well-behaved daughters, aged 12 and 10. However, they experienced annoyance and despair with the behavior difficulties of their 9-year-old hyperactive son, Joel. When the teacher complained about their son's behavior, detailing his distractible style of learning and describing his emotional outbursts, Mr. and Mrs. A. felt extremely pressured and helpless. Mr. A. repeatedly stated that he and his wife just didn't know what to do with their son, despite their usual feeling of being very resourceful persons, who cope efficiently with their daughters' difficulties (especially in academic areas). Now, Joel's parents expressed the fact that they bitterly resent their feelings of helplessness. The consultation began with the psychologist focusing the discussion on Mr. and Mrs. A.'s interpersonal skills to deal effectively with their son's expressions of anger.*

Cole (1986) exemplified the interplay between demands and resources. Resources include individual, familial, and community support systems that serve to minimize the impact of the stressors and to reduce the probability that the family will enter into crisis. The picture that emerges from parental reports among parents of disabled children constitutes one of extraordinary demands for time investment and on the physical, financial, and emotional resources of every member of the family (Mullins, 1987). The severity of the children's difficulties may be related to increased levels of family distress, while an adequate support system can counterbalance the accumulation of family stresses. Gallagher, Beckman, and Cross (1983) reported that higher levels of parental stress have been associated with the child's slower rate of progress, more difficult temperament, less social responsiveness, and the presence of additional care-giving demands.

Mothers of handicapped children have often expressed their fatigue, viewing themselves as chronically exhausted. Cohen and Waren (1985) reported that these mothers often become a therapist, teacher, trainer, and transporter. They further noted that the responsibility for caring for the disabled child is often made heavier by tasks given to parents by specialists, and by the need to transport the child to various settings for specialized medical care. All of these tasks should be considered important, but to perform all of them is cumulatively overwhelming and does not allow the same amounts of free time and freedom of role choice as have mothers of nonhandicapped children.

*Case study: Ron L.'s mother*

*Ron's teacher was surprised when his mother, Mrs. L., began crying on parents' day at school. Ron, a 7-year-old learning disabled boy, had several special education needs and received the help of the resource teacher in school. In addition, Ron's mother transported him to several types of after-school remedial treatments, such as remedial reading, speech therapy instruction, and a music enrichment program. On parents' day, after acknowledging the amount of help and support that Mrs. L. already provided her son, the teacher had suggested that it would be very helpful if the mother would also tutor him and provide help in a new school project. Mrs.*

*L., through her tears, shared with the teacher her feelings of unease and ambivalence. She wanted to help her son and to find an answer to all his needs, but she also had to care for her other children. Being the children's transporter, teacher, and mother, Mrs. L. felt extremely tired and burdened by an overload of duties, not having any time left for herself. She explained to the teacher that she felt trapped by the teacher's suggestions for additional new duties and roles. Although she sincerely wished to be involved in Ron's education and to foster his growth, Mrs. L. already felt she did not have any free time left and doubted the wisdom of taking on more responsibilities which she believed may have a negative impact on her ability to continue to function.*

Parents' expectation from themselves -- to become their children's educators and therapists -- has raised special concerns that this may place further stress on families who could already be overloaded by the demands of everyday living with a disabled child (Short-Degraff, 1987), affecting the parents' ability to perform their main roles as fathers and mothers.

## Stress and resource interrelations

Early research found correlations between the number of life stressors and the probability of stress-related illness (Holmes & Rahe, 1967), but recent evidence indicated that stress-related distress should not be predicted on the basis of quality and quantity of stressors alone. Rather, predictions should include examinations of other variables that moderate the potential deleterious effect of the stressors (Peterson, 1984).

McCubbin and Patterson (1983) emphasized the importance of the family's definitions of: (a) their stressors and handicapping conditions, (b) their available and needed resources, and (c) the power and flexibility of their coping for reorganization and change in order to meet the new demands. Parental stress has been associated on the one hand with the special characteristics of the child (e.g., the severity of the handicapping conditions and the presence of additional behavior and health problems) and on the other hand, with the types of social support available to the family (Gallagher, Beckman & Cross, 1983; Margalit, Shulman, & Stuchiner, 1989).

Peterson and Wikoff (1987) demonstrated that at least three adjustment variables are related to raising a handicapped child: maternal health, marital adjustment, and a subjective assessment of the problem. The adjustment variables as a whole are related to the number of problems brought about by the handicapped child and to the resources available to the family. The greater the number of stressors, the greater the problem in marital adjustment and maternal health.

In turn, the family's coping resources and functioning are likely to be mediated by the ecological systems (Bronfenbrenner, 1979; 1986) within which they must interact and be acted upon, such as schools, centers, agencies, etc. Factors that may exacerbate feelings of stress, and factors that may serve a stress-resistance role in mediating or buffering the stressful events have been the focus of investigation (Holahan & Moos, 1985). The consistent but rather modest correlations found in the research between life stress and psychological distress or symptomology (Avison & Turner, 1988) suggests the important role played by mediating factors which may buffer the stress' influence.

Peterson and Wikoff's (1987) analysis indicated that not all families with high stressors experience adjustment problems. These results proposed that the study of moderating variables which immunize or buffer an individual from the negative consequences of stressors, such as disease and interpersonal dysfunction, should be emphasized in stress research. Resources available to the individual and the family may help reduce the potentially deleterious outcome. Such resources may include personality variables, social support, coping skills, and family climate. However, it should be emphasized that these factors are not necessarily mutually exclusive: Family climate can be considered both a supportive social network and a resource in buffering stress, whereas both coping style and social support may be viewed either as resources or as personality variables. Various aspects of personality should be the focus of attention in order to further determine the parental roles and needs among families with mildly disabled children.

## Personality variables

Major research attention has focused on personality variables that may operate as personal resources during stressful periods (Johnson & Sarason, 1978). Three phases of any stressful event can be defined:

1 The initial reactions to the disruptive event (i.e., the representative phase).
2 The cognitive evaluation of the event.
3 The person's activities toward reducing the interference of these reactions.

Regarding the first phase, research has indicated that individual characteristics play a primary role in one's initial reactions to stress. For example, stress has been related for some individuals to somatic symptoms and complaints (Hendrix, Steel, & Schultz, 1987). Others may feel depressed and tired. With regard to the second and the third phase, the personality disposition underlying the related variables of self-efficacy, self-confidence, and perceived control is especially relevant. Bandura (1982) explained that perceived self-efficacy concerns judgments of how effectively one can execute courses of action necessary to deal with situations involving stressful elements. Summarizing a series of studies on the stress-resistance process, Bandura concluded that the self-efficacy construct predicts a wide range of adaptive life-behaviors, including coping behavior.

Rosenbaum (1987) proposed that three personality repertoires affect the person's coping style, emphasizing their central role in predicting coping strategies: sense of coherence (Antonovsky, 1979; Antonovsky & Sourani, 1988), hardiness (Kobasa, 1979), and learned resourcefulness (Rosenbaum, 1987).

### Sense of coherence

The sense of coherence comprises a global orientation that expresses the extent to which one has a pervasive, enduring though dynamic feeling of confidence that: (a) the stimuli deriving from one's internal and external environments in the course of living are structured, predictable, and explicable;

(b) the resources are available to meet the demands imposed by those stimuli; and (c) these demands are considered as challenges, worthy of investment and engagement (Antonovsky, 1979). Antonovsky (1979, 1987) defined the sense of coherence as consisting of three interrelated components:

Comprehensibility
Manageability
Meaningfulness

The person with a high sense of comprehensibility expects the stimuli that he or she will encounter in the future to be predictable, or at least, when they come as a surprise, to be ordered and explicable. The manageability component refers to the available resources that may be either under one's own control or controlled by others whom one feels that he/she can trust and rely upon. Individuals who have a high sense of manageability will not feel victimized by unexpected events. The third component, meaningfulness, refers to emotional perspective within the construct, highlighting the importance of being involved. The meaningfulness component serves as the representative of the motivational element in the coherence construct (Antonovsky, 1987).

Individuals with a high sense of coherence usually consist of those who evaluate stressors in a more positive way, because they feel generally confident that their internal and external environments are predictable, that a high probability exists that things will work out as well as can be expected, and that they feel emotionally involved in many areas which are viewed as worthy of effort investment.

## Hardiness

Hardiness may be considered to be another personality construct that can be positively related to effective coping with stress. From the existential perspective (Maddi, 1976), Kobasa (1979; 1982) proposed the existence of a hardy personality style. Kobasa (1979) defined hardiness as consisting of three interrelated components:

Commitment
Control
Challenge

Commitment may be defined as the ability to believe in the importance of truth and interest value, and to have an overall sense of purpose in life. Committed individuals tend to involve themselves in whatever they are doing, rather than performing in an alienated, perfunctory manner. They feel curious about their environment, involve themselves in their activities, and interpret the events they experience as meaningful.

Individuals with control orientation feel and act as if they are influential in the face of life events through their use of knowledge, skill, and choice. Hardy people, in this respect, believe that they can shape their fate, and reject the notion that luck, chance, or unfriendly powerful others may determine it. A sense of control leads to actions directed toward transforming events so that they fit into the individual's overall life plan.

People who view life as a challenge believe that change rather than stability is normal and that change presents opportunities for growth. Persons who welcome challenge are characterized by openness, flexibility, and tolerance of ambiguity. Similarly, it is expected that hardy individuals will emphasize the positive and desireable aspects of most life situations (Kobasa, 1979; Kobasa & Puccetti, 1983).

## Learned resourcefulness

Any effort at coping with stressful events involves attempts at self-regulation (Rosenbaum, 1987). Learned resourcefulness (Rosenbaum & Ben-Ari, 1985; 1986) has been defined as a personality repertoire consisting of a set of behaviors and skills by which individuals self-regulate internal responses that interfere with the smooth execution of an ongoing behavior, using self-control methods during the action phase.

Sense of coherence, hardiness, and learned resourcefulness all constitute personality repertoires that may have stress-buffering effects, yet each of them has the potential to mitigate the effects of the stressful events at different phases of the self-regulation process. Hardiness and sense of coherence are postulated to influence the person's evaluation of the stressful disruption (i.e., the primary appraisal of the stressor), whereas learned resourcefulness is postulated to influence the person's actions toward reducing the interfering effects of one's emotional reactions to a stressor, rather than the primary appraisal of the stressor (Rosenbaum, 1987).

Holahan and Moos (1985) added another perspective to the personality variables that play a critical role in stress regulation. They identified the people who were able to adapt to stress without experiencing physical or emotional strain, and found that they were more easygoing in their interpersonal style, and tended not to keep their feelings of strain bottled up, nor to express them antagonistically in interpersonal relationships.

## Social support

Social support has been consistently related to stress research, and has been hypothesized to serve as a buffering mechanism, mediating the effects of stressful events (Cobb, 1976; Crnic, Greenberg, Ragozin, Robinson, & Basham, 1983; Haggarty, 1980; McCubbin, 1979; Peterson, 1984; Unger & Powell, 1980). The individual's belief in the existence or availability of people on whom that person can rely for care, value, and love, seems a critical stress-mediating factor (Mitchell, Billings & Moos, 1982; Sarason, Levine, Basham, & Sarason, 1983; Schmidt, Conn, Greene, & Mesirow, 1982).

Social support, which constitutes an important link between the social environment and the psychological well-being of individuals in stressful situations (Vaux, 1987; Vaux & Wood, 1987), may serve as a central resource to the family with a mildly disabled child. Social support is usually defined as the information leading the individual to believe that s/he is cared for, loved, esteemed, and a member of a network of mutual obligations (Cobb, 1976). Two basic elements comprise social support: (a) the number of available others to whom individuals believe they can turn in time of need, and (b) the degree of satisfaction they anticipate from the available support from these persons (Sarason & Sarason, 1986).

### Types of support

Unger and Powell (1980) distinguished between support from formal (e.g., physician) and informal (e.g., neighbor) sources. They reported that families use different types of support to meet different needs, and that a context specificity exists which determines the differential use of support networks. These types of supportive resources may address different needs among the stressed individuals, yet the role of these various types of support cannot be conceptualized as distinct or exclusively different. Kazak (1987) emphasized the heterogeneity of supportive social networks available to families with disabled children, demonstrating that only an individualistic approach, which attempts to study the significance of the different networks as related to familial needs, will provide a meaningful answer to the critical question of which aspects of social networks reduce the stress faced by these families.

Cohen and Wills (1985) identified four types of resources afforded by social support:

Emotional
Informational
Companionship
Material

*Emotional support* comprises the expression of feelings that a person is well regarded and valued. Usually this type of support is provided by informal sources of support such as friends and family members. *Informational support* involves providing advice intended to help a person understand his/her predicament within a formal setting. When the person needs additional information necessary for decision making or problem solving, the information may be provided as a means of support by people whose knowledge in the needed area is regarded as reliable, such as professionals and experts.

*Companionship* refers to spending time with others in leisure or recreational activities. In order to avoid feelings of loneliness, companionship support is valued and provided in an informal manner by friends and family members. *Material* support constitutes the provision of financial and material resources or the provision of actual assistance toward completing a task. This type of support can be provided by community agencies in a formal style, or by friends and family relatives in an informal style. Often substantial intercorrelations exist between the measures of the different dimensions, while at other times, relatively little correlation is found between them.

Cohen and Wills (1985) hypothesized that the different types of social support elicit different effects on feelings of stress. Emotional and informational support were found to exert a more widely beneficial impact than tangible aid. By lessening the threat to self-esteem or self-efficacy posed by negative events, emotional support thus has a more generalized effect. Similarly, informational support causes a reappraisal of the negative events in ways that reduce their stressfulness. On the other hand, instrumental support and social companionship were expected to have a positive influence only in very specific situations, primarily when the coping resource complements the source of stress (for example, monetary assistance will mainly tend to alleviate financial distress).

## Individual differences in parental needs

Research has demonstrated that parental needs for social and professional support are varied and include: more opportunities for social networks and interactions, free access to professional information and advice, and access to extra-familial resources. Mental health professionals and special education personnel play an important role in monitoring familial and individual needs and in providing appropriate services, but only if these workers develop an individualistic approach in their comprehensive planning (Burden & Thomas, 1986; Cirillo & Sorrentino, 1986).

It is accepted that individual differences exist in the need for contacts with others and in the personal meaning attached to these contacts (Sarason, Sarason, Shearin & Pierce, 1987); in addition, self-efficacy appears to be related to social support. People with low levels of social support, or with dissatisfaction from the support available to them, may not believe that other people are interested in them. Sarason, Sarason, Hacker, and Basham (1985) found that individuals who differ in social support provoke different reactions from others. People who describe themselves as low in their number of social supports are also less favorably evaluated by the subjects with whom they interact than are those with a high range of social support. Social competence has often been associated with a high level of social support.

Implicit or explicit in much of the research on social support rests the idea that social support comprises an environmental provision -- "something" that the individual "obtains" from interpersonal relationships. However, growing evidence suggests that the person's perceived social support level functions as a stable attribute over time, has traitlike characteristics, and can be viewed as dependent on individual differences or as a general aspect of interpersonal relationships (Sarason & Sarason, 1986; Sarason, Sarason, Shearin, & Pierce, 1987). In order to be helped, the person must possess certain characteristics, needed both to gain and to maintain interpersonal relationships (Sarason, Sarason, Hacker, & Basham, 1985).

## Support and well-being

The impact of the different types of social support upon well-being is also related to personality differences (Hill, 1987). The interrelations between mood and social interrelations exemplify this area of study. Brandstatter (1983) found a significant relationship between mood and social interrelations: Subjects' mood was better when they were interacting with other people, and thus felt socially supported, rather than when they were alone.

In Clark and Watson's (1988) study, the high association between positive mood and participation in social events was strongly confirmed; however, the direction of this cause-effect relationship remains unclear. Is engagement in social activities likely to be emotionally uplifting, as the person experiences the social support (whereas staying alone at home leads to depressed feelings), or does an elevated positive mood generate greater social interrelation, enabling the person to feel supported socially? The negative depressed mood often reported among parents of disabled children (Wikler, Wasow, & Hartfield, 1981) may be caused by their belief in their loneliness, reporting lower levels of social support available to them, but on the other hand, the negative mood may also comprise the reason for the parents' lower abilities to perceive available social support and to develop meaningful social interactions. These relations seem interactional and transactional in their nature.

Another personality variable related to social support consists of the person's need for affiliation. Hill (1987) identified two distinct types of support -- material support and socioemotional support -- and found that these two types were differently related to well-being, depending on the individual's affiliative need levels (i.e., individuals with a high affiliative need level tend to benefit from more instrumental types of support). Individual differences in personality structure must be considered in order to meet the different needs for social support among parents of disabled students.

## Conclusions

This chapter explored factors related to rearing a disabled child which contribute to increased feelings of stress, and factors that serve as buffering mechanisms which mediate the effects of stressful life events. Family definitions of their stressors, resources, and abilities to cope with the demands of the handicapped child have been considered central to the family members' adjustment. One mechanism by which support may promote adaptation lies in its impact on coping processes (Fondacaro, & Moos, 1987). For example, the provision of information or advice by a significant other can have a direct influence on coping behavior. Indirect influences include the effect of emotional support on enhancing an individual's self-esteem and sense of self-efficacy, which, in turn, may facilitate the ability to access and enact coping strategies. Several personality characteristics were viewed by researchers as playing an important role in the functioning of parents with handicapped children, such as the sense of coherence, hardiness and learned resourcefulness. Each personality construct has emphasized several cognitive and emotional features that play a critical role in successful coping. However, a central role in the stress, resources, and coping paradigm has been given to social support.

Research reported different types of social support, such as emotional, informational, companionship, and material, which have different impacts on the stressful feelings of individuals. For example, social support has also been found to be more beneficial to the recipient when it facilitates a sense of self-efficacy and control over one's environment. The impact of the different types of social support upon the individual's well-being is also related to individual differences. However, the direction of the interrelations between personality differences and availability of social support is not clear. The research results reflected constant interactions between these variables, which cannot be viewed within a cause-effect model. Social support does not constitute an objective resource available within environment, but rather more resembles a trait within the individuals themselves that enables them to benefit from resources available within their community. The family can be considered one of the most important sources of social support and the central link in any support network. As such, the family environment deserves further exploration, with the goal of evaluating parental abilities in the context of the resources and other facets of the family climate affecting each of the family members.

# 6
# Family Climate

The family climate concept has special importance in the understanding of family systems with mildly handicapped children. Family social climates can be portrayed according to the interpersonal relationships among the family members, the directions of the personal growth which are emphasized in the system, and the family basic's organizational structure. The study of family climate using Moos' conceptualization (1987a, 1987b) represents a comprehensive approach to investigating, on several dimensions simultaneously, the life situation as defined by the shared perceptions of the family members. Moos highlighted the importance of the three dimensions composing the family climate construct: *Relationship, Personal Growth, and System Maintenance* (Moos, 1987b).

> The *Relationship* dimension is measured by the Cohesion, Expressiveness, and Conflict subscales, assessing the extent to which people are involved with and supportive of one another, and the degree of commitment, help, and support family members provide for each other. Information is also provided by this dimension regarding: the extent to which family members are encouraged to act openly and to express their feelings directly; and the amount of openly expressed anger, aggression, and conflict among the family members.
>
> The *Personal Growth* dimension is measured by the following subscales: Independence, Active-Recreation, and Achievement, Moral-Religious, and Intellectual-Cultural orientations. These subscales evaluate the underlying goals toward which the family setting is oriented. They assess the extent to which the family members are assertive, make their own decisions, and are self-sufficient. This dimension depicts the extent to which activities are cast into an achievement

oriented or competitive framework; as well as the degree of family interest in social, intellectual, cultural, recreational, and religious activities.

The *System Maintenance* dimension includes the Organization and Control subscales, providing information about the order and the structure of the family, the clarity of expectations, the degree of openness to change that characterizes the family, and the extent to which set rules and controlling procedures are used to run family life.

The Personal Growth dimensions channel the direction of change within the family system, while the Relationship and System Maintenance dimensions influence the individual's commitment to the family environment, as well as the extent of possible system change and of personal costs involved (Moos, 1987a; 1987b).

## Family environment and child adjustment

Understanding family climate can provide insight into the role of the family system in child and adolescent development. Study of the origin of children's social competence has progressed along two parallel paths. One path has been followed by researchers who have focused on the quality of family relationships and early experiences, and the other by those who have focused on social problem solving skills and information processing patterns. In Pettit, Dodge, and Brown's (1988) survey, a hostile, inconsistent parenting style was found to predict the development of aggressive behavior and social incompetence in children. Conversely, socially competent behavior with peers has been predicted by warm, responsive parenting within the family environment.

In a survey of studies identifying associations between family environment and adolescent adjustment, Moos (1987b) conceptualized that adolescent development is promoted in families that encourage independence and provide modeling for instrumental and social skills, whereas in families that emphasize achievement in a context of conflict and accommodation to restrictive rules, adolescent development is hampered (Moos, 1987b).

Many studies have linked aspects of family environment to children's cognitive development. Whereas a warm, supportive family climate tends to foster natural cognitive development, an overly rigid achievement orientation can inhibit it. More generally, family climate influences mental development because better family relationships increase the level and the quality of the stimulations provided for the child (Moos, 1987b).

Cornell and Grossberg (1987) found that families of gifted children were higher in Cohesion and Expressiveness, indicating that family members place great value on mutually supportive relations and open expression of thoughts and feelings in the family. These families scored high on both Active-Recreational and Intellectual-Cultural orientations, but somewhat surprisingly low on Achievement orientation. It would appear that these families value recreational and intellectual pursuits, but not in the context of an achievement-oriented or competitive framework. Finally, these families scored low on Control, reflecting a relative lack of emphasis on set rules and procedures in the family life.

In Cornell and Grossberg's (1987) study, the importance of the Relationship dimension was emphasized, viewing the quality of the family interaction as critical to the child's adjustment. They concluded that the most important factor for the child's adjustment and personality development consisted not of *what* parents do with their children, but *how* they do it. A cohesive family relationship and lower levels of family conflict were associated with children's overall adjustment, fewer problems with discipline, and more favorable cognitive development and school achievement. Family expressiveness has been associated with better adjustment scores of the children, higher self-esteem, and lower anxiety.

Children's behavior difficulties were also found to be related to aspects of family climate. Children in poorly organized families tended to be more maladjusted and impulsive. Many hyperactive and aggressive children have been found to be from families which demonstrated high levels of conflict and low levels of cohesion and expressiveness (McGee, Williams, & Silva, 1984; Moos, 1987b). Gil, Keefe, Sampson, McCaskill, Rodin, and Crisson (1987) found that the Independent/Organized levels of the family environment were related to predicting symptom severity among children. Higher scores on the Independent/Organized factor were related to fewer symptoms, whereas higher scores on the Moral/Religious factor were associated with more symptoms. It can be concluded that Independent/Organized families may buffer against the effects of stress.

Special attention should be focused on the climate variables in families with handicapped children. The need to identify the optimal mix of individuals' interactions within a setting will help in planning effective interventions to structure optimal environmental climates for promoting personal growth and adjustment (Moos, 1987b).

## Climate in families with a disabled child

Consistent trends have been identified in several studies with regard to the family climate among families with mildly disabled children. The presence of a handicapped child in the family seemed to affect the family climate, and has been found in several studies to be related to a decrease in the social activities of the family members, lower levels of open expression of feelings, less cohesiveness between the family members, and an increased structuring of the family activities (Margalit & Heiman, 1986; Margalit & Raviv, 1983). It can be concluded that in these families a clear tendency exists for a more rigid climate and for less support, either internal (i.e., levels of cohesion and acceptance of free expression of feelings) or external (i.e., social activities and interrelations outside the family).

Parents of learning disabled children demonstrated conflict avoidance behavior, which resulted in less conflict resolution, overprotectiveness in their interrelations, and increased rigidity (Margalit, 1982; Margalit & Heiman, 1986). These parents also reported higher levels of anxiety, with an increased emphasis on the system-maintenance and personal growth dimensions of their family system. In contrast with families of mentally retarded children, where parents are often confronted with the clear and consistent difficulties of their children, and tend to decrease their familial expectations for achievements and personal growth (Margalit & Raviv, 1983), the parents of learning disabled children seemed to exhibit confusion, anxiety, and a need for personal compensations.

*Case study: Gil P.*

*Gil's parents complained about their son's behavior difficulties in the school and home settings alike. As a hyperactive, learning-disabled boy, he was easily distractable, often bored, quarrelsome, and easily getting into trouble. Mr. and Mrs. P. asked for psychological consultation from the school psychologist, as they felt ineffective as parents and anxious to introduce change into the family climate.*

*The assessment of the family climate, using the Family Environment Scale (Moos, 1987b), substantiated the information provided through the interview, yet pinpointed attention at specific aspects in need of intervention. Relatively high levels of familial conflicts were reported, although the family members did not provide encouragement to each other to express their feelings openly and freely. Both parents felt supported within their family system, with the mother viewing the family system as more cohesive than did the father.*

*Mr. P. viewed himself as a highly ambitious and intellectual individual who greatly valued his personal independence, and he judged the present family situation as a threat to his personal freedom and independence. Mrs. P. accepted the family's uncomfortable circumstances, in which she was less able to protect her independence or her intellectual striving, but she revealed far more concern with aspects of the family interrelationships. Mrs. P. was more annoyed by the family's quality of relations, and especially with the conflicts between the family members. Both parents reported that they almost did not have time or personal energies for leisure activities.*

*The mother openly emphasized the importance of the family's order and structure, viewing it as a necessary condition for Gil's functioning. She felt that if the rigid order within the home environment were not maintained, their son would demonstrate additional difficulties and expressions of maladjustment. She believed that her son felt more secure in a structured and ordered environment, with clear rules and expectations. Both parents were dissatisfied with the present solution to their son's distractibility tendencies. Both Mr. and Mrs. P. were worried that the rigid climate within the family could foster Gil's compulsive tendencies. They already noticed that he was currently less able to tolerate changes at home, and even at school. However, Mrs. P. accepted this typical family climate as a necessity, to decrease the child's distractibility, whereas Mr. P. constantly attempted to introduce flexibility and changes into their lives.*

The brief case study demonstrated the impact of the boy's distractibility and hyperactivity on the family climate dimensions, increasing the need for structuring the family environment, and decreasing the spontaneous expressions of emotions. The mother's independence, personal ambitions, and intellectual aspirations were also affected, as a result of the overload of her caring duties for her son.

## Families living in the kibbutz environment

In an attempt to isolate the sources of stress and to investigate resources and coping variables, the family climate of handicapped children in the Israeli kibbutz has been studied. The kibbutz as an independent economic community provides its members with an equal and sufficient supply of food, housing, clothing, physical space, recreational outlets, and medical care (Kaffman, Sivan-Sher, & Carel, 1981), and the kibbutz also maintains comprehensive social plans (medical, retirement, and disability insurance programs). Active participation and involvement in the community's decision making process is accomplished through an extensive system of social institutions, including the general assembly which is the supreme body, and a network of committees.

The role of childrearing in the kibbutz has attracted the attention of psychologists, sociologists, and educators. The ideological foundation underlying the communal childrearing practice was detailed by several authors (Beit-Hallahmi, 1981; Bettelhiem, 1969; Gerson, 1978; Rabin & Beit-Hallahmi, 1982). Communal education comprises all spheres of the child's life, including physical, cultural, educational, and health care, and is organized into age groups from birth through late adolescence. Kibbutz children live and often even sleep in children's houses, spending several hours in the afternoon in their parents' homes.

In this child-centered community, where the children are economically dependent not on their parents, but rather on the community, and where resources are provided according to personal needs, the normal daily parental duties, as well as the additional daily caring for the disabled child, are minimized through the communal food preparation, laundry services, and childrearing arrangements. In such a community, the emotional impact of having a disabled child, in terms of the family climate, has special theoretical significance.

## Family interviews

In order to acquire qualitative data on the unique nature of the parental experience among kibbutz families with a disabled child, and to validate the assumption that the kibbutz constitutes a unique situation in which the increased demands and overloads were controlled, semi-structured interviews were used in the first stage of the research series, in order to gather information on 102 families of disabled children who reside in 47 Israeli kibbutzim throughout the country. Half of the sample's disabled children slept in communal housing arrangements, and the other half slept in family-based arrangements (Leyser, Margalit & Avraham, 1988).

The interview results demonstrated that parents of disabled children appreciated the specific support and increased amount of resources that the kibbutz life made available to their families. Almost all parents pointed out that the kibbutz provides for all the educational, medical, rehabilitational, and recreational needs of the child with special needs. Some of them even said that although at some time they had considered leaving the kibbutz due to various personal reasons, the kibbutz's support regarding their present economic needs, as well as the daily care of the child available only in the kibbutz community, influenced their decision not to leave. Several parents talked appreciatively about the very expensive services received by their children, such as medical evaluations and therapies performed by well-known experts, both inside and outside the kibbutz, and even abroad. Furthermore, the daily management of the child and his/her routine caregiving were provided by the system, enabling both parents to continue working.

Parents often mentioned that they were highly grateful for the social support and understanding available to them by fellow workers at their workplaces. They reported almost no difficulties in receiving release time from work, whenever a need arose to accompany the child or to participate in any diagnosis or treatment (e.g., medical, educational). The parents also related that they have many friends in the kibbutz, and that they continue to participate in various social events. Yet, some mentioned that they must take turns attending these social events, so that during the children's visits to their parents' homes, one of the parents can stay to monitor the disabled child, while the other participates in the community event.

However, ambivalent feelings regarding the kibbutz social structure were expressed, possibly as a direct result of the strong emphasis in the kibbutz ideology on the precept that each kibbutz member possesses equal privileges and obligations. Parents wanted the kibbutz to accept and provide for their special needs, but they did not wish to emphasize that they were not an ordinary family with needs equal to those in every other family in the kibbutz. They felt it was important that their fellow kibbutz members would view them as any other ordinary, equal, and "normal" family in the community.

The emotional impact of having a disabled child was especially reported by these parents. They expressed the pain of having a disabled child, accentuating their concerns with regard to the uncertain future waiting ahead for their disabled child. These findings substantiated several other studies that reported such anxiety as the major concern for parents of disabled children (Wikler, Wasow & Hartfield, 1981). However, this uncertainty was not expected to be expressed in the present study, as the kibbutz is similar in many ways to an extended family, providing for full social security within a life-cycle perspective. In contrast to the researchers' expectations, most kibbutz parents did report their most significant concern as related to their children's future, and they disclosed their apprehension that the disabled child may become a burden on his/her nondisabled siblings.

This concern may be regarded as a universal expression of continuous stress and of fear of the unknown. These parents, despite the kibbutz environment, felt anxious with regard to their present key role in monitoring the lives and welfare of their disabled children, and to the threat of future loss of control.

Some families expressed ambivalence with regard to their social interrelations. As mentioned above, they reported having many friends in the kibbutz, yet they emphasized their profound feelings of loneliness. Social support was readily available to them in the kibbutz environment. Friends expressed interest in the special child's progress, and many times offered their assistance.

However, parents reported that they needed more concern and empathy, not only for themselves as parents and for the child's well-being, but also for themselves as human beings. Several families even pointed out that despite their many social connections, they felt that they did not have any "real" intimate friends in the kibbutz. These expressions of subjective distress and loneliness are similar to those documented among parents of disabled children outside the kibbutz. It can thus be assumed that these feelings of uniqueness and social isolation are not a function of overwork in order to acquire the additional resources necessary for raising a disabled child, but rather are a reflection of the emotional pain and distress experienced by parents with disabled children everywhere.

In summary, on the basis of the parental interviews, it can be concluded that the availability of utilitarian resources and community support was viewed by these parents as an extremely important resource for coping. However, several major sources of distress remained: (a) the constant need to monitor and demand additional special services for the disabled child from the community; (b) the deep concern regarding the child's future; and (c) the loneliness, social isolation, and feelings of uniqueness as related both to the children's interrelations with their peer groups, and to the parents' interrelations with the other kibbutz members.

## Family climate in the kibbutz

The results of these interviews were further supported by the findings from the family climate research in the kibbutz environment. In this environment, where the increased financial, medical, educational, recreational, daily caretaking, and other objective resources necessary for attending to the disabled child's greater needs are provided by the community, a unique opportunity exists to study the emotional, subjective impact of the disabled child on his/her family, when the increased objective burden is controlled. Based on the assumption that the presence of the disabled child in the family may introduce systemic changes in such an environment, a series of studies (Leyser, Margalit, & Avraham, 1988; Margalit, Leyser, & Avraham, 1988; Margalit, Leyser, Avraham & Lewy-Osin, 1988) was executed on families of disabled and nondisabled children, with regard to their family climate and confidence in their world.

These studies attempted to investigate in what ways the availability of various resources accessible to individuals in the kibbutz may or may not function to buffer stress and promote adjustment (Margalit, Leyser, Avaraham, & Lewy-Osin, 1988). They found that even within this extremely supportive community network, tuned in to the individual needs of its members, parents of disabled children expressed a lower personal sense of coherence and less satisfaction from their family life, and they reported a different pattern of family climate. They viewed their families: as providing less support; as enabling less close interrelations between the family members; and as recognizing the existence of greater, unresolved conflicts within the family system.

It is unclear whether the greater conflicts resulted in the family members' attempts to separate themselves from one another and to lower their expectations for a cohesive and supportive family climate; or whether the emotional distancing within these families led to their increased conflictual interrelations. Although the kibbutz provided these parents with resources similar to those provided to other parents for promoting their personal growth, the parents with disabled children felt less able to use these opportunities for recreational and intellectual pursuits in comparison to other kibbutz members. Families of disabled children reported that they were less free to devote time to intellectual-cultural activities or to other leisure activities. They emphasized their feelings of decreased freedom and independence, as compared to the other members in the community. They felt less able to invest resources in their personal growth, resulting in an arrest in family and personal growth.

## Conclusions

The different aspects of family climate reflect an important dimension in the understanding of functioning in families with disabled children. Family climate dimensions have been found to be related to children's academic performance and behavior adjustment. The more intensive, committed, and socially integrated a setting, the greater its potential impact becomes, especially on personal factors that are changing developmentally. Some emphasis on each of the three family climate dimensions (relationships, growth, and maintenance) facilitates positive social and performance outcomes, but too much focus on any area can have problematic consequences. Too much emphasis on personal goals, for example, can lead to anxiety and stress in the family. Cohesive, homogeneous settings tend to influence incongruent individuals to change in the direction of the majority, whereas a heterogeneous setting has more diverse influences and provides each person with a wider choice of options.

The results of the studies reviewed, in line with the conceptualization of social support, demonstrated that various aspects of family climate are affected by the presence of a disabled child. The family system often loses some of its supportive abilities, enabling less freedom of emotional expression, and less opportunities for personal growth. A frequent emphasis on rigidity and structural dimensions creates a family system which lacks some of its abilities for growth and change. Attempted intervention programs which provide appropriate, individually adapted resources may help parents to cope better with their immediate increased needs. However, the kibbutz study demonstrated that providing resources according to needs may help parents to cope better with the organizational aspects of their prolonged stress, but not with the emotional strain of parenting a disabled child. Even in the kibbutz environment, where all resources are provided by the community, the pain and sorrow of these parents cannot be ignored and should be particularly acknowledged. The results demonstrated that support should be provided not only to address the immediate day-to-day needs of these parents and to facilitate the development of their children, but also reflecting the consideration that the life-cycle of these individuals has been affected and that their opportunities for personal growth may be endangered.

Adequate support must attempt to empower these parents in strengthening their coping skills and feelings of control, and the planning of such supportive interventions must consider individual needs, including those resulting from gender differences.

# 7

# Fathers' and Mothers' Roles in the Family

Within the family context, social support and family climate variables have been linked in different ways to coping among men and women. Caring duties have often been considered as the mothers' major role among families of disabled children, whereas fathers tended to assist mothers in their overload of duties, thus identifying themselves as mothers' helpers. This division of responsibility between the sexes may be in part a function of gender-related differences, but obviously, strictly traditional sex-roles are no longer the norm in our society. In the current discussion, mothers and fathers will be compared and contrasted, but the reader should keep in mind that each parent in reality takes on the most personally relevant and appropriate role, regardless of traditional distinctions. The entrance of computers into the homes of disabled children enables the development of a new parental role -- in support of the home-computing performance. This chapter aims to investigate fathers' and mothers' roles and preferences within the family, with the goal of identifying new roles adapted to sex differences.

## Parental response as a function of gender differences

The increased caring duties among mothers of disabled children heighten these women's vulnerability to the effects of stress, as reflected in their greater complaints regarding feelings of fatigue and symptoms of ill health. Compared with other mothers, mothers of handicapped children spend more time on child-care and housework and receive less reinforcements for their efforts (Schilling, Schinke & Kirkham, 1985). Fathers reported fewer symptoms of distress, higher self-esteem, more internal self-control, and less need for social support (Goldberg, Marcovitch, MacGregor, & Lojkasek, 1986).

Special consideration has been devoted to families of children with mental retardation and behavior disorders (Margalit, Shulman & Stuchiner, 1989), in which fathers and mothers were found to react differently to the psychopathology of their children. For fathers, both types of psychopathology -- the externalized and the internalized disorders -- seemed to be related to their feelings of stress, whereas mothers' stress seemed to be related mostly to externalized disorders. It may be assumed that for fathers, expressions of aggression and acting-out seemed as threatening as the demonstrations of behavioral isolation and anxiety manifestations. Mothers, who usually provide most of the caring and controlling of the disabled child, expressed more distress as related to the child's externalizing behavior disorders.

## Gender differences in family climate perceptions

The mothers' profiles of their family climate reflected that they were more affected by the family crisis than were the fathers (Margalit & Heiman, 1986). Mothers of mentally retarded and learning disabled children viewed their family climate as less encouraging of open and free expression of emotions, and as less enabling of independence and recreational activities for the family members (Margalit & Raviv, 1983). The mothers' special emphasis on organization and control within the family system may be viewed as an efficient coping behavior for stressful and anxiety-provoking situations. This increased structuring and controlling within these families should not be considered as related to hostile and negative feelings, but may rather be viewed as suitable to the greater needs of these children for order and structure in their environment.

For parents, family climate variables have been related to stress, yet in a different manner for mothers and fathers. Limited opportunities for personal growth predicted increased stress for fathers, whereas the existence of support within the family, in terms of closer relations between the family members, served to buffer the mothers' feelings of stress. With regard to general feelings of stress, the interactions between family climate variables and children's psychopathology explained a large proportion of stress for mothers and only a small proportion for fathers (Margalit, Shulman & Stuchiner, 1989).

The comparisons between the kibbutz fathers with and without disabled children revealed that they differed in their sense of coherence, and in their personal growth opportunities. The kibbutz provided fathers of disabled children with resources for all their material needs, attempting to prevent the role organization crisis that is conceptualized as a direct function of the increased demands on the family resources. However, fathers' emotional reactions remained pronounced. Fathers of disabled children perceived fewer opportunities than their peers for every aspect of personal growth. They felt that they were less free to develop personal independence within their family systems, and they also reported having less opportunities for both types of personal growth activities: intellectual-cultural activities, and active-recreational pursuits.

These findings require further investigation, in light of the fact that the analysis among fathers in the disabled children's group revealed that the personal growth measures were highly and significantly correlated with the sense of coherence. The correlational nature of the analysis did not enable a conceptualization of a directional explanation: It is unclear whether the fathers' lower coherence left them with less personal energy to invest in themselves, or whether they perceived less freedom to invest in themselves and fewer opportunities for personal growth, which led to their lower coherence. It should be further emphasized that the kibbutz community provided the two groups of parents with similar opportunities for intellectual and leisure activities, yet fathers of disabled children were less able to benefit from these opportunities.

Mothers of disabled children in the kibbutz also reported having a lower sense of coherence and felt less satisfaction from their familial life. They viewed their family system as less supportive of cohesive relations, and as more emphasizing of conflictual interrelations. Similarly to fathers, they also viewed their families as less enabling them to participate in intellectual-cultural activities, yet in other aspects related to personal growth, such as independence and leisure activities, they did not feel differently from mothers of nondisabled children.

## Gender differences in social support

The adequacy of social networks has predicted adjustment for both fathers and mothers of handicapped children (Frey, Fewell, & Vadasy, 1989). However, Holahan and Moos (1985) found that family support operated as a stress resistance factor differently for women and men. Women tended to deal with stress by turning to other people for support, whereas men tended to respond to stress with social withdrawal (Shaw, 1982), and to use cognitive coping and problem solving strategies focused on a search for instrumental solutions to realistic child-care problems.

Sarason, Sarason, Hacker, and Basham (1985) found that women were evaluated as more skilled socially, and reported greater perceived social support and greater satisfaction with the support available than men. However, fathers were less preoccupied than mothers with negative or depressed mood and were better able to respond creatively to challenging parental tasks (Frey, Fewell, & Vadasy, 1989). Kobasa and Puccetti (1983) suggested that the role of the family support for men may be more complex: For male executives low in hardiness, family support was found to be detrimental to health. Kobasa and Puccetti speculated that for these individuals, family support engendered inappropriate coping with stress in the workplace. Presumably these gender-related differences are the function of conventional patterns in sex-role behavior in our society: the individualistic, instrumental reactions of males to stress, as compared with the interpersonal and cooperative reactions of females (Schilling, Schinke & Kirkham, 1985).

Cronkite and Moos' (1984) results suggested that women may be more attuned to social supports than are men, and that lack of support is especially related to the use of ineffective coping strategies among women. Women who reported more family support relied less on avoidance coping and showed less depressed mood than women with low levels of family support. This pattern of results was not observed among men. Wives' and husbands' social networks differ in several aspects. Wives draw on strong network ties (typically close friends and family members), whereas husbands' support systems tend to be less intimate and are weighted with work associates (Schilling, Schinke & Kirkham, 1985; Tognoli, 1980). However, the meaning and structure of optimal support for men should be studied in depth, and the potential sources of support that may be strongly related to coping and adjustment among men (such as support from co-workers) have not been examined. Family support was more strongly related to functioning among women, whereas work support was more strongly related to functioning among men.

In line with the vast research findings suggesting that women usually cope with stress by turning to other people and usually view social support as their major source of assistance, for kibbutz mothers the personal interrelations within their family systems were the best predictor of their personal coherence. Kibbutz fathers, on the other hand, emphasized the role of personal growth opportunities as the critical factor for their sense of coherence.

## The personal growth perspective

The fathers' reports of limited opportunities for personal growth have a special meaning within the stress-coping paradigm. Their personal growth opportunities were consistently related to the sense of coherence and well-being of fathers, affecting the life-cycle development. Fulfillment of personal ambitions for growth and independence were especially emphasized as important by fathers. It appeared that their decreased opportunities in the city were attributable to greater demands on the family resources; however, the kibbutz study demonstrated the inadequacy of such a conceptualization of the situation. It cannot be attributed to the lack of material resources related to the disabled child's greater needs. Fathers on the kibbutz objectively had access to the same free time and financial resources as in the other families. However, they reported a decrease in their independence and less freedom or time to devote to intellectual-cultural or recreational activities, resulting in an arrest in personal growth.

It is not clear whether these fathers lack the emotional resources necessary to invest in their own well-being due to their personal distress, or whether they fail to emphasize their personal growth because of the dynamics in the kibbutz society. Although the communal philosophy of the kibbutz movement requires that every member contribute to the system according to his/her capacities, and that every member be provided for according to his/her needs, these fathers are acutely aware of their children's consistently greater needs. In this situation, they may feel uncomfortable asking the kibbutz for additional resources for their children and may avoid using other resources (i.e., for themselves) whenever possible, in order to be considered a normal family.

## Development of the father's unique role

A growing body of literature on father-child interactions demonstrated that fathers have a unique and significant effect on their children (Clarke-Stewart, 1978; Lamb, 1977). Fathers have traditionally been viewed as responsible for transmission of competent, instrumental, problem solving behavior (Frederick & Wellborn, 1988). Research has demonstrated that the children of "involved" fathers were reported to have self-regulative styles, adaptive strategies, and capacities for achieving school success.

In comparing perceived father versus mother involvement, both parents were found to influence children's perceptions of competence and autonomy. However, perceived father involvement was found to be related to boys' perceived competence, whereas mothers' involvement was not (Frederick & Wellborn, 1988). The father-child relationship is jeopardized when the child is handicapped (Vadasy, Fewell, Meyer & Greenberg, 1985). Gallagher, Beckman, and Cross (1983) highlighted the special role of fathers in these families and the need for its comprehensive study. Reviewing the critical question of whether there exists a unique male role to be played in the family of the handicapped child, the need for intensive research in this area was emphasized, calling for the conceptualization of an active and unique paternal role in families of handicapped children.

However, in several studies of family climate, fathers seemed to lose their unique perspective in the family climate (Margalit & Heiman, 1986). The differential parental roles to be played by fathers and mothers in assisting the computerized activities of their mildly disabled children deserve further exploration. In order to achieve the expected advantages from the introduction of computers at home, the intervention program should aim to reinforce the unique gender-related parental role through parent-child-computer interactions.

## Conclusions

Family climate and social support variables were found to be differentially related to stress for mothers and fathers in different environments. Mothers of disabled children have evidenced higher vulnerability to the effects of stress than have fathers. In line with their general tendency toward other-oriented coping strategies, mothers showed more sensitivity to and need for social support, especially in the family. Fathers, who tend to respond to stress by social withdrawal, revealed a greater need for personal growth opportunities. The delineation of a unique role for the fathers of disabled children should constitute the focus of active efforts in further research and intervention. It should be emphasized that, although mothers currently play the primary role in caring for their disabled children, individual differences between family configurations continually remind us that fathers may also take on the major childcare role and mothers may adopt more instrumental functioning. Research tends to generalize sex-role differences, despite the fact that in our progressive society, both men and women are breaking down stereotypical barriers. The types of assistance and intervention needed by these parents consist of those which empower parents of disabled children in their coping efforts, attuned to differential parental needs.

# 8

# Empowering Families: Effective Interventions

Professionals who offer assistance to those in need, do so in the hope that it will produce both immediate and long-term positive consequences. However, substantial evidence has now been accumulated suggesting that different types of help, and the manner in which they are offered, can have either empowering or usurping consequences, depending upon the intertwining of a host of intrapersonal and interpersonal factors (Dunst & Trivette, 1987).

## Empowerment

Empowerment, which can play a crucial role in the ability of a family with a mildly disabled child to support the child's computer-assisted and other activities, may be viewed from a social systems perspective. The following three basic aspects underlie this perspective:

1 *Proactive stance*: People are already competent, or have the capacity to become competent.
2 *Enabling experiences*: Opportunities are created for competencies to be displayed by the social systems.
3 *Control*: The person who needs help must attribute behavior change to his or her own actions in order to acquire a sense of control.

These three aspects provide a basis for viewing empowerment from a broader-based social systems perspective that emphasized the importance of the parents' subjective evaluations of the situation, and the help-giver's behavior as part of both enabling and empowering families. The computer's entrance into the homes of disabled children may help provide enabling experiences, that will emphasize not only aspects of personal growth relevant to the disabled child, but also a growing climate for all the family members. However, individual differences between parents should also be considered, as related to developing opportunities for exposure to enabling experiences, and regarding the capacity to feel competent within the family environment.

The goals of effective interventions for empowering families should include providing parents with greater access and control over needed resources. Toward that end, these parents can be assisted to improve their decision making and problem solving abilities through proper training. An additional instrumental behavior that is necessary for parents to acquire consists of the capacity to interact effectively with others in order to procure resources.

Special attention should be focused on the help provider as the source of help-giving. Various forms of help-provision may create positive or negative effects on parental empowerment. For example, some types of help-giving are likely to foster dependency. Somewhat ironically, the more supportive and positive the help-giver is, the more likely dependency may occur. If the help does not require the help-seeker to acquire effective behavior, the immediate needs of the person may be met, but passivity and dependence will increase, and the ability to learn effective behavior will diminish. Help-giving may also elicit negative reactions if incongruence or a mismatch exists between what is sought and what is offered.

Help-giving may produce learned helplessness if it undermines the family's competence and control. This is likely to occur when help directly reduces the help-seeker's control over life events and reactions to them; prevents or interferes with the acquisition of new competencies; interferes with the perceived self-efficacy of the help-seeker; conveys a sense that s/he is inferior or incapable of solving problems; or creates situations where credit for successful outcomes is attributed to the help-giver rather than to the help-seeker.

The parents' coping style plays a major part in their responsiveness to empowering interventions. Only a differential investigation of coping strategies among mothers and fathers with handicapped children may guide the developing of new models to empower these parents.

## Coping strategies

Understanding the coping strategies of fathers and mothers with handicapped children may play an important role in directing their intervention planning. Coping can be defined as cognitions and behaviors used by the individual in evaluating the cognitive and emotional meanings of stressors, and in initiating activity to decrease the impact of stress, in order to reduce or manage anxiety and other distressing emotional states (Folkman & Lazarus, 1988). In their transactional model of stress and coping, Lazarus and Folkman (1984) identified problem solving and regulation of emotions as the two major coping functions, either of which may be expedited in one or several of the following four ways:

Information seeking
Direct action
Inhibition of action
Intrapsychic processes

The relation between emotion and coping in stressful encounters has been conceptualized as bidirectional, with each affecting the other. Each of the four coping strategies is perceived as either oriented to the self or to the environment. The appraisal and coping process is thought to play an important role in moderating the effect of stress on well-being (Lazarus & Folkman, 1984; Moos & Billings, 1982). The appraisal process generates emotions that influence the coping processes, which in turn change the person-environment relationship. The altered person-environment relationship is reappraised, and the reappraisal leads to a change in the quality and intensity of emotion (Folkman & Lazarus, 1988).

### Paradigms for coping strategies

A common characteristic of many coping taxonomies has been the distinction between more active or approach strategies (i.e., active confrontations of the stress' source, including behavioral efforts to deal with challenges and cognitive attempts to manage one's appraisal of the stress), and strategies that rely essentially on avoidance of the problem (i.e., efforts to deny, minimize, or escape the stressful situation). Approach coping strategies such as information seeking and problem solving have been positively related to adaptation, whereas avoidance coping strategies have been negatively related to adaptation (Holahan & Moos, 1985; Kobasa, 1982).

Holahan and Moos' (1985, 1987a) comprehensive research in coping strategies was not able to identify a single strategy as critical for successful coping. However, processes of cognitive appraisal and attributions which correlate with perceptions of control have been viewed as stress reducing, and an active, instrumental, problem-focused coping style was considered more adaptive than were avoidance strategies (Holahan & Moos, 1987b; Litt, 1988). Especially interesting is the finding that approach coping failed to discriminate between healthy and unhealthy groups of individuals (Holahan & Moos, 1985). Thus, when faced with life stress, most individuals engage in high levels of approach coping, with an addition of some avoidance coping. It is this additional amount of avoidance coping that distinguishes between adaptation and maladaptation. Pearlin and Schooler (1978) reported that coping strategies involving selective ignoring exacerbated rather than reduced stress in the areas of marriage and parenting.

Problem-focused or emotion-focused forms of coping are associated with a change in emotions (Folkman & Lazarus, 1988). These coping forms can be problem solving oriented (i.e., attempting to achieve an environmental change), and/or intrapsychic, inner-directed (i.e., attempting to regulate emotions and to change attitudes, cognitions, and emotions concerning internal demands and conflicts related to the stressful event) (Friedrich, Wilturner, & Cohen, 1985). It should be noted that coping efforts which modify the environment are appropriate only when the environment lends itself to change. In circumstances beyond the individual's control, intrapsychic coping may serve to regulate affect and to facilitate adaptation. Processes of cognitive appraisal and attribution which correlate with perceptions of control have generally been viewed as stress-reducing (Litt, 1988). A paradigm for the different types of stressors, resources, and coping strategies is illustrated in Figure 8.1.

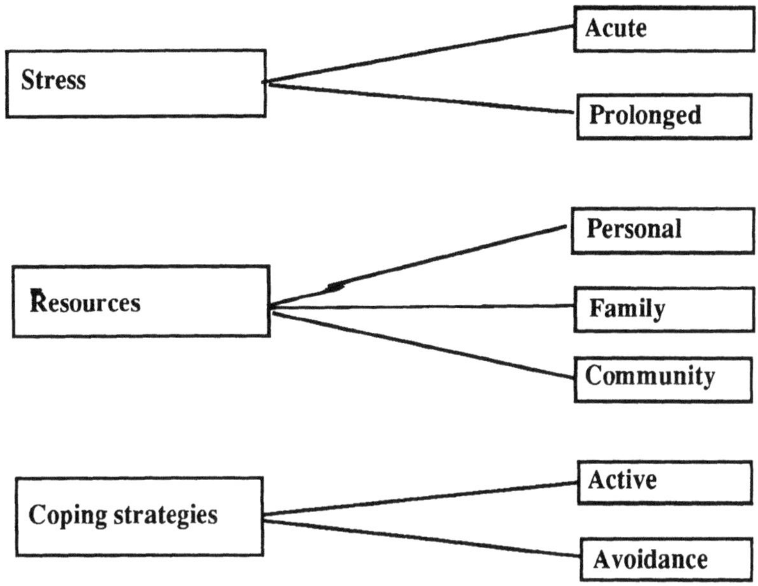


Figure 8.1. Stress, resources, and coping paradigm

Problem solving as a coping action can be understood by examining the interactions among several factors (Heppner & Krauskopf, 1987):

1 The characteristics of the particular problem.
2 The four major problem solving processes: Encoding; goal setting; developing plans and pattern matching; and taking action.
3 A host of individual differences or personality variables which affect how people process information during problem solving.

According to this model, a problem consists of a situation in which individuals may respond in relation to their internal or external demands. Inherent in this definition lies the subjective perception of the problem, and problem solving is possible only when the person perceives at some level that a response is required.

Coping strategies have been studied in terms of generalized tendencies reflecting the personal style of the individual, or as context dependent, reflecting the specific characteristics of situations and conditions (Folkman & Lazarus, 1980, 1985; Friedrich, Wilturner, & Cohen, 1985). It follows that although their coping style reflects their individual differences, parents in families with mildly disabled children may also demonstrate similar coping tendencies that stem from their shared family context. The characteristics of this family ecology thus deserve further discussion.

## Conclusions

Individuals are profoundly affected by the social matrix in which they are embedded (Moos, 1987b). As parents have the capability for promoting their mildly handicapped children's growth, and in light of the realization that these parents' life-cycle is affected and their opportunities for personal growth may be endangered, the goal of comprehensive interventions for empowering these parents should consist of helping them develop coping skills attuned to their individual needs and personal style. The appraisal of available resources and coping strategies may change the person-environment relationship. Coping theories emphasized the bidirectional relations between emotion and coping. Two types of coping were discussed: problem-focused and emotion-focused. Coping was examined as a primary factor in the parental response to empowering interventions.

The critical connections between the family environment and its children's school-related attitudes and performance, among disabled and nondisabled children alike, emphasize the value of developing a model to plan the parental role for assisting children's computerized activities at home. Families can amplify the impact of school, reinforcing school achievements, or families can compensate for the lack of impact, as when they teach skills at home that children do not learn in school. Cohesive, supportive, well-organized families tend to promote students' adjustment and scholastic skills.

An educational intervention comprises but one of the multiple life contexts and specific settings that influence personal growth and maturation (Parkerson, Lomax, Schiller & Walberg, 1984). Other powerful current environments also shape development, mood, and performance. Thus, by inhibiting and augmenting their effects, or by compensating for their lack of effect (Moos, 1987b), family environment can alter the outcome of educational programs, such as programs in the area of computer uses for mildly disabled students. Through an intervention model which reinforces unique parental roles and trains fathers and mothers to introduce and support computer-assisted interventions for their disabled children, a greater benefit can be expected from the entrance of technology into homes.

Consultation programs, in order to be effective, should emphasize parental life-cycle perspectives, focused on aspects of their sex roles: instrumental aspects of facilitating personal growth among the fathers of mildly disabled children, as well as the interrelational aspects of facilitating familial and extrafamilial support among the mothers. Mothers and fathers differ in their coping strategies and in their perceptions of children's needs, and especially in their own sense of responsibility for providing these needs. In this section, personality variables, social support and family climate have been examined in terms of the stress, resources, and coping paradigm for the study of family ecology in families with mildly disabled children. Parental attributions and familial contexts have a crucial role in the child-computer interactions, as will be presented in Section 3.

# Section III

## The Entrance of Computers into Families

# 9
# Parental Expectations

The literature survey presented in the first section of this text demonstrated the possibilities for empowering disabled children through computer integration into their education. The use of computers has been recommended not only to facilitate the children's learning at school, but also as a means of creating a bridge between schools and homes, and of fostering parental involvement in their children's education (Epstein, 1985). Technology's rapid entrance into the education of disabled children was shown to be directly linked to the advantages for these children of computer integration into their schools. The research survey demonstrated several advantages of computer integration for disabled children in various academic areas, yet pinpointed attention on the importance of structured, strategic instruction which is firmly rooted in sound cognitive and curricular theory in each of the recommended areas.

The advantages of computers' home availability for these children was related to extending time to experiment and develop important skills, thus increasing the opportunities to foster the children's development. However, this simplistic model of children's support through the computer's presence in the home allows for only a partial understanding of the phenomenon. The simple provision of technology was not found to result in any significant changes for the children's achievements; consequently, the role of the significant adult (i.e., a teacher or a parent) was emphasized as critical for the effective integration of computers either at school, or in the student's home.

The review of the research on parental stress, resources, and coping strategies in the second section of the text revealed an additional perspective for the understanding of family dynamics, with implications for parental abilities to provide meaningful support for their handicapped children. In light of the crucial role attributed to significant adults in computer integration, it follows that the parental attitudes toward the computer, the reactions to its introduction into the home, and the home-school interrelations deserve central consideration in order to facilitate the development of effective, supportive father and mother functioning as related to home-computing. Chapter 9 aims to render an in-depth exploration of home-school interrelations and of parental expectations from technology, as related to their children's specific needs which initiate parental stress. Results from a recent survey of 80 fathers and mothers with disabled children (Margalit, Rochberg, & Greenberg, 1988) will be presented in order to demonstrate the importance of the parents' expectations, and the sources of their stressful feelings will be analyzed with the goal of enhancing the understanding of parental functioning.

In social learning theory (Bandura, 1978), people are viewed as playing an active role in creating their information generating experiences as well as processing and transforming informative stimuli that happen to impinge upon them. This involves reciprocal transactions between thoughts, behaviors, and environmental events. The predictive value of reciprocal consequences derives partly from people's expectations of how their actions are likely to change future consequences. The development of an effective parental support model for children's home-computing requires the study of parental beliefs about action-outcome contingencies, as well as the meanings that parents attribute to (a) their present stressful situation, and (b) possible outcomes from computer usages.

## Cognitive appraisal of parental stress

The theory of psychological stress and coping developed by Lazarus and his colleagues (Lazarus & Folkman, 1984) emphasizes the value of cognitive appraisal as one of the critical mediators for stressful person-environmental relations. Cognitive appraisal constitutes a process through which the person evaluates whether a particular encounter with the environment is relevant to his/her well-being (Folkman, Lazarus, Dunkel-Schetter, Delongis, & Gruen, 1986). The study of parental appraisal regarding those aspects of their stressful feelings which are related to their disabled children's special needs may facilitate the development of intervention plans to foster parents' coping strategies and their children's future adjustment. Parental beliefs regarding the expected advantages from home-computers will be meaningful only if they are relevant to the sources of parental stress which are related to the children's difficulties.

## Parental stress related to areas of children's adjustment

Handicapped children's adaptation obviously constitutes an area of concern for their parents, and a distinction can clearly be made between the children's current difficulties, which create problems for the family members in the present, and the children's prospects for future adjustment in society, over which parents may agonize and worry. In the study of 80 fathers and mothers with disabled children, the parents considered several areas, representing a balance between current and future considerations, as extremely important and as worthy of resource investment. Two-thirds of the parents (N = 54, 67.5%) considered their children's future ability to reach independence in adulthood as a major source of stress, and the children's future vocational opportunities were also mentioned by 45 of the parents (56.3%) as an important source of anxiety. Aspects of their children's current functioning which were related to parental stress were also identified: Stress and anxiety was emphasized by 37 parents (46.3%) in relation to their children's leisure activities; 34 parents (42.5%) viewed the children's learning difficulties as a major source of stress; and 34 parents (42.5%) pinpointed their children's social difficulties as a major concern. These parents clearly revealed that areas related to the consideration of their children's future opportunities were perceived as more stressful than were their children's current difficulties.

### *Stress from current leisure activities*

An interesting aspect of these parental attitudes consists of the similar proportion of parents who expressed emotional involvement and concern for each of the three areas of current difficulties, with an emphasis on the leisure activities as creating even more stress than the learning and social difficulties. This finding was consistent with the interviews, where parents often described their irritation stemming from their children's difficulty in effectively using their periods of free time. The following case studies portray some aspects of the difficulties inherent in disabled children's leisure activities.

*Sara T.: A busy daughter and desperate mother*

*Mrs. T. described her mixed feelings of concern, anger, and guilt regarding her 12-year-old learning disabled daughter. The extremely tired mother (after a full working day) felt annoyed that her main role consisted of being a transporter to various remedial teachers and to several organized art activities available for children at the local museum. The mother complained bitterly that most of her afternoons were dedicated to her disabled daughter and that the planning and initiating of all of Sara's afternoon activities were the mother's duty. Mrs. T. felt guilty at her anger, yet could not help her feelings of desperation, knowing that whenever her daughter had a few free minutes, she would approach her mother, asking "I am bored, I don't have anything to do; What shall I do now?" Sara was unable to become involved in television programs for more than a few minutes at a time; she was unable to occupy herself in any self-initiated play activity; and she was completely dependent upon her mother's suggestions and constant assistance.*

*Gal M.: A lonely boy*

*Another mother, Mrs. M., explained that she was emotionally prepared for the learning difficulties of her 7-year-old mildly mentally retarded son, and took comfort in the knowledge that Gal received academic support from a professional teacher. However, the focus of her difficulties in dealing with her son revolved around Gal's behavior during his free time periods. Mrs. M. felt that she could not cope with Gal's constant nagging about his feelings of boredom and loneliness. During Gal's leisure time, his mother was repeatedly reminded of the limitations of his disability and the differences between her son and other children.*

Disabled children's passive life style and dependence on adults for planning leisure activities (Margalit, 1984) seem to constitute a source of parental stress in similar proportions to that related to learning and social difficulties.

Additional areas of importance which were also mentioned by several parents, but which parents regarded as having a lesser impact on stressful feelings, consisted of the children's health difficulties, discipline problems, and moody behaviors. In light of these children's mild disabilities, it is not surprising that health difficulties did not constitute a major area of concern. It also seems that these parents did not experience major discipline problems with their children.

## Expectations from computers

Schaefer and Edgerton (1985) emphasized the importance of parental attitudes and beliefs for predicting children's development and for planning intervention programs. Rokeach (1968) stated that attitudes and beliefs predispose the individual to respond in some preferential manner. In order to investigate the meaning of the computers for parents with disabled children, the 80 fathers and mothers surveyed were asked about their beliefs regarding the critical areas in which computers could potentially help their children.

The analysis of these expectations from computers (see Figure 9.1) revealed that 55 parents (68.6%) viewed the computer as an important answer to the children's leisure needs, and 52 parents (65.0%) expected the computer to be an important source of assistance for the children's learning difficulties. Only 39 parents (48.6%) expressed the belief that the computer could greatly expand the children's vocational opportunities, and 24 parents (30.0%) expected a strong impact on the children's future independence. The entrance of computers into the home was expected by 22 parents (27.5%) to significantly affect their children's social difficulties, and 23 parents (28.8%) even believed the computer would demonstrate a profound impact on their children's emotional adjustment and moodiness.

It can be summarized that parental beliefs related to home-computing of their children seemed to be closely related to

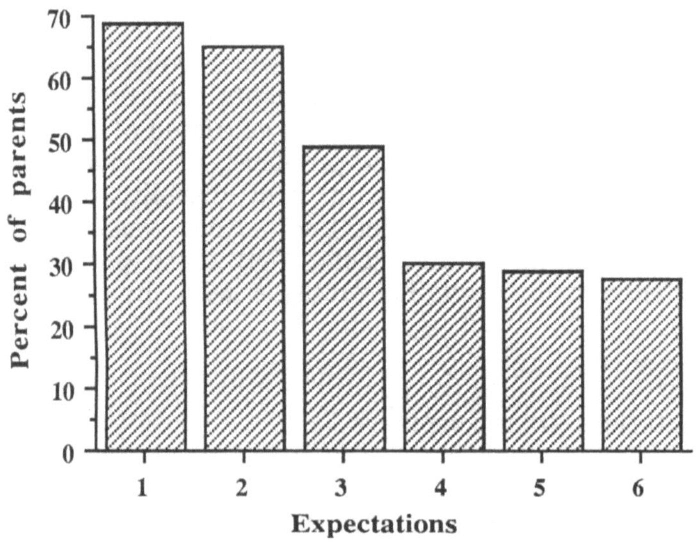


1 - Leisure
2 - Learning
3 - Vocational opportunity
4 - Independence
5 - Emotional stability
6 - Social interrelations

Figure 9.1. Parental expectations from computer integration

their major sources of worry and anxiety, especially regarding current areas of expectations, and to a lesser extent with respect to future considerations.

The results of this study substantiated Naisbitt's (1984) conceptions about the ubiquitous trap of people believing, or more accurately, hoping, that technology will solve all their problems, and thus, to some extent, abdicating their personal responsibility. Parental excitement and eagerness to introduce computers to their disabled children may represent the parents' desire to believe that technology stands on the verge of liberating them from their overloaded personal burden. In their tense, overworked, and emotionally distressed state, many parents of disabled children may convince themselves that computer technology will reduce parental responsibility in fostering their children's adjustment and will in fact solve most of their problems. These beliefs should signal professionals to evaluate the danger of parents' over-expectations regarding the anticipated "magical" effects of the computer.

In the process of intervention planning, such parental attitudes cannot be ignored, as they will likely serve as a source of parental disappointment and anger when the computer fails to live up to their high expectations. Awareness should particularly be maintained regarding the emotional atmosphere surrounding the computer's entrance into the home, an atmosphere tinged with elation and exaggerated hopes. In order to avoid anger and disappointment, which may render fathers and mothers emotionally incapable of supporting their children's computer efforts, parents in the early stages of computer introduction must be continually reminded that, although powerful, the computer possesses no magical effects. Computers may foster children's development only if parents develop a more realistic set of beliefs, viewing technology not as a means of reducing parental responsibilities, but rather as an additional remedial tool in which the parent-child interrelations, rather than the child-computer encounters, constitute the focus of interest. Indeed, the importance of parental involvement throughout the process of computer integration into both home and school must be repeatedly accentuated by intervention workers, in order to reinforce parental involvement even prior to the purchase of the home-computer.

## Sex roles

In order to further investigate parental beliefs regarding the computer's promise, the sex role aspect was studied. Fathers' and mothers' differing attitudes toward stressful aspects of their children's functioning and expectations from computers have potential for complementing and supplementing one another during the process of home-computer introduction.

## Stress-related areas of child adjustment

In the study of the 80 parents (Margalit, Rochberg & Greenberg, 1988), several gender differences were revealed by the comparison of the 36 fathers' and 44 mothers' perceptions, regarding areas of difficulty related to parental stress. Of the fathers, highest levels of concern were reported with regard to their children's future independence (N = 28, 77.8%), and as related to the future vocational opportunities available to their children (N = 23, 63.9%). Mothers also emphasized the tension induced by these two areas of concern for the future, yet in more moderate terms. Of the 44 mothers, 26 (59.1%) viewed their children's independence in adult life as their highest area of concern, and 22 (50.0%) emphasized stress related to their children's limited vocational opportunities.

With regard to current sources of stress, 61.1% (N = 22) of the fathers were very concerned with leisure activities, in comparison with only 34.1% (N = 15) of the mothers. More mothers (N = 21, 47.7%) were highly concerned with their children's learning difficulties, whereas only 36.1% (N = 13) of the fathers viewed this area as a major source of stress.

The results of the study emphasized the importance of future planning as a major source of parental anxiety for both sexes. Fathers and mothers alike were primarily concerned with their children's abilities for achieving independence in adulthood, and secondly were concerned with the vocational opportunities available to their children in the future. The differences between fathers and mothers with respect to their disabled children's future adjustment were related to the proportions of parents of each gender experiencing that stress. Fathers more than mothers expressed higher levels of concern in these areas. With respect to areas of current functioning which evoked tension, fathers were more highly concerned about their children's inability to spend their free time in an enjoyable and independent manner, whereas mothers evidenced more concern regarding their children's learning difficulties.

## Expectations and coping patterns

The comparison of the fathers' and mothers' beliefs regarding the computer's advantages for their children development revealed that fathers expected more than mothers that the integration of computers could help their children in their most important areas of difficulty. Among the parents, most of the fathers (N = 29, 80.6%) and more than half of the mothers (N = 26, 59.1%) believed that the computer usages would introduce a significant change into their children's free time. Another important area, in which a large proportion of both fathers (N = 26, 72.2%) and mothers (N = 26, 59.1%) held strong beliefs, was that the computer would significantly assist the children in dealing with their learning difficulties. Some of the fathers surveyed even expected computers to help with their children's health difficulties, an area that none of the mothers surveyed found applicable to computer solutions. The fathers' higher levels of expectations from computers corroborated research on male coping styles and on the subjective meaning of computers for the male members of the family. The study of parental coping strategies revealed that males' coping preferences were often found to be more instrumental, and the fathers' expectations from the computers support this notion. Mothers, on the other hand, preferred two types of coping: Interpersonal coping, such as receiving support from others, and Avoidance coping where an attempt was made to avoid direct confrontation with and excessive worry due to the source of difficulty.

## Social and subjective differences

Males and females were found not only to differ in their general coping strategies, but also in their social and communication patterns about computers. Whereas computer involvement implies potential isolation from social contact, for many male members of the families surveyed, the computer helped increase social associations through game playing. In some families, the father and son spent hours together at the computer. Moreover, many males seemed eager to share their computer expertise with others, and became enthusiastic about teaching theoretical and technical aspects. In a study of 526 high school students (Remp, 1985), similar patterns were evidenced. More male students reported that they contacted peers for advice on the computer. Female students reported talking about computers equally to men and women, whereas male students reported that four-fifths of their contacts were male.

Males have also frequently been found to articulate their enthusiasm, appreciation, and special relations with the home-computer. In Bauer's (1988) study, a clear gender difference emerged in the ways that men and women expressed their subjective experiences of the computer. Turkle (1984) explored aspects of the "subjective computer" and how people view it. Using Turkle's notions, Bauer (1988) identified the differing male and female metaphors, suggesting that the "male" computer had a playful or recreational quality (a toy), whereas the "female" computer was utilitarian (a tool that did or did not have a practical application). Women viewed computers primarily as technological tools, whereas the men more readily saw its expressive potential, and in many instances established a personal connection to it. In addition, many women were resentful, estranged, and primarily anxious about the computer usage.

The computer interactions for the mothers often seemed to have a particularly threatening impact on the women's sense of competence. As a result, in several families, mothers were not actively involved in supporting their children's computer interest. They typically did not (or could not) play the role of a teacher, tutor, or playmate in relation to their children's computer interest, unlike some fathers who played games with, assisted, or even wrote special computer programs for their children. Bandura's (1977) concepts of self-efficacy add an important explanation to this situation. The fear to learn to use computers, which several mothers expressed, greatly influenced their willingness to engage in such a task, as well as their efforts and their persistence in maintaining the process.

The survey's results clearly demonstrated the potential of the new instrument to enhance father-child interrelations, fostering a new and unique role for fathers. Fathers' positive attitudes toward computers suggest the potential to reinforce their ability to support their disabled children in an area viewed as an enjoyable activity. However, these results also alerted the planner to a potential difficulty. The fathers' enormous hopes for significant improvement and their strong beliefs in the value of the technology for their children's present and future development are liable to lead to frustration and disappointment. Parental counseling should attend to these two aspects, facilitating the realization, albeit frustrating, that the computer's potential will not reduce parental responsibilities and overload, but rather may enable parental involvement with their children's activities in an area that is appealing to fathers and children alike.

Two additional aspects in the development of models for mothers' and fathers' involvement should be considered: (a) individual differences between parents, and (b) parent-school interrelations.

## Individual differences

The interviewed fathers, as a group, expressed more positive attitudes towards the computer usages. They seemed more excited than the mothers, expressing more global positive beliefs and a greater readiness to invest time and effort into home-computing activity. However, as individuals, a varied range of belief and expectation patterns emerged among the parents interviewed. Several brief descriptions of the detailed case studies collected (Margalit, Rochberg & Greenberg, 1988) may exemplify the heterogeneity within and between family systems, pinpointing the different parental roles evident in these ecological settings.

### *Mr. and Mrs. D.: Computer users at the office*

*In the D. family, both father and mother expected a profound change through the entrance of the computer into their home, with regard to the achievements of their 10-year-old learning disabled daughter who suffers from severe reading difficulties. Both Mr. and Mrs. D. work in banks, and had already been exposed to computers at their workplaces. During the interview, Mrs. D. was generally supportive of the idea of computer integration, but her husband revealed far greater enthusiasm. Mr. D. emphatically pointed out his daughter's improved academic performance as a result of using her home-computer. He praised her new and more effective communication style, and he even remarked that his daughter even seems more beautiful to him now.*

*David B.: Father and son sharing an interest*

*Mr. B., a technician, was extremely excited to introduce technology into his home in order to help his 5-year-old learning disabled and hyperactive son. He was certain that everyone would be surprised by David's abilities to concentrate on one task for a continuous period of time. Mr. B. was prepared to devote time to his son's efforts with the computer, and even contacted several friends, attempting to identify appropriate software. Mrs. B., a housewife, seemed more reserved in her expectations, appeared very tired and annoyed by her son's acting out and disruptive behavior, and expressed her wish that through the computer the father and son would develop closer relations. She complained that her husband's current impatience with their son's restless behavior resulted in an emotional distance between David and his father. The parents reported that the father often became annoyed and angry at his son's behavior, and Mr. B. expressed the hope that "... now with the computer everything will be different. The boy will be able to concentrate for longer periods of time, and I will enjoy helping him with interesting software."*

*Mr. and Mrs. H.: Inexperienced users*

*Mr. H., an accountant, and Mrs. H., a lawyer, reported that despite their university education, they did not have any prior knowledge regarding computers, and they both felt anxious and reluctant about its introduction into their home. However, in this family, the mother expressed higher expectations from home-computing for their 10-year-old mentally retarded son, whereas the father seemed more reserved. Both parents had shared the decision to purchase their home-computer, and they were currently seeking guidance and support.*

The study of parents' interviews emphasized the need to avoid group generalizations in preference of an individualized, multidimensional model of parental involvement in the home-computing activities of their children. The study of parent-school interrelations further emphasized the different styles of parental involvement in the integration of computers within their children's educational settings.

## Home-school connections

In order to study the processes affecting the nature of children's home-computing and technology-related home-school connections, two major forces must be considered (Giacquinta & Lane, 1988):

1 *School leadership*: The degree to which teachers invite, encourage, and emphasize the importance of parental involvement and home-school interrelations in the area of computers.
2 *Parental leadership*: The degree to which parents assist with their children's activities.

The interplay between school and home requires a partnership between these two settings. It seems obvious that neither partner should be ignored in effective technology integration, and that parents who reveal an interest in becoming active in their children's schoolwork should especially be encouraged. However, research has indicated that such an attitude toward parent involvement has not typified the schools.

### Survey of home-school relations research

Recent research in nondisabled children's computer usage has indicated that, although most of these children were engaged in educational microcomputing in their school settings, parents and teachers seldom worked together to promote such activities at home (Edyburn & Lartz, 1987; Epstein, 1985). Although it was generally accepted that schools should carefully consider the possible contribution of home-computers to classroom learning, only a few schools have attempted to coordinate these activities with homes (Epstein, 1985).

A study of home-computing interrelations among parents and children of 51 families of nondisabled children (Levin, 1988) demonstrated that on the one hand, these parents did not perceive a need to become involved in their children's educational microcomputing efforts at home, and that, on the other hand, the children's school did not work toward creating a need for parental involvement or opportunities for home-school integration. As a result, the use of computers at home by nondisabled children was found to be completely separated from its uses at school, and some parents even conditioned the use of computers at home to fixed times during the week, or postponed its usage until after schoolwork had been completed, saying that the computer is intended for "fun" while the schoolwork is "serious" (Levin, 1988).

Most children in Levin's (1988) study were not using their home-computers for academic learning, although there was some utilization of the computers for word processing and for programming. Neither children nor parents seemed aware of how their home-computers might be used to expand on school learning. Many parents were not knowledgeable enough about academic microcomputer activities to realize that it may have been necessary for them to become involved in such activities, if they wanted their children to engage in them. In addition, the schools have not been helpful in making parents aware of how computers at home can be used to support and enrich classroom work.

## Home-school relations for disabled children

In several special schools and classes in Israel, a wide gap was found between formal and informal school-home connections related to the computers. Headmasters and teachers, during meetings at Tel Aviv University's School of Education, reported that parents, and especially fathers, were active and helpful during the first stages of the computer's entrance into the schools. These fathers assisted schools in finding resources for acquiring hardware and software and aided teachers in operating the new technology whenever a difficulty was met. Teachers thankfully reported that even fathers who seldom tended to visit the schools and who often expressed complaints and dissatisfaction with the system, were rather enthusiastic in their offering of help and demonstrated appreciation of the role of the new technology integration in their children's education and rehabilitation process.

However, most of the parents' activity was performed in the school environment, by fathers who had prior technological knowledge, experience, and skills. Of special interest was the fact that teachers highly appreciated and encouraged such parental assistance. They gratefully accepted parental suggestions and did not feel threatened by these encounters. Yet, it should be emphasized that these teacher-parent interactions were mostly directed toward increasing the effectiveness of computer integration into the schools, not into the homes.

Parental needs for counseling and support were almost ignored in the area of increasing the effectiveness of the home-computing of their children and selecting educational software to serve as a bridge between their children's learning activities in the school and home environments, and to compensate for the special educational needs of these children.

Many families with disabled children already owned computers in their homes, yet parents were rarely advised in a planned manner with regard to guidelines for computer usage, in order to help their children, and with respect to increasing the cooperation between school and home practice. Many parents did not even know in what manner and in which areas their children were using computers at school. The parents expressed a desire to help their children's effective use of computers at home and a need for assistance and guidance.

In the few schools where teachers did provide parents of disabled children with the information about the software used in the classroom, it was found that this had been initiated by the students or the parents, and not by the teachers. In two families, although they owned computers for a considerable period of time, the disabled children were not using them. Parental reports did not clarify whether the children were not allowed to use the computer, or whether they were unsuccessful in the family competition for computer time, developing attitudes of helplessness.

One of the children, an 8-year-old male student with learning disabilities, asked for parental help in acquiring time on the family computer, explaining that the teacher gave him homework on the mathematics drill-and-practice software used in school. He also invited the parents to see him working, eager to demonstrate his skillful performance. Another learning disabled adolescent brought software home to teach his younger brother the keyboard skills that he had learned and mastered at school, thus "earning" his family computer time. These children's attempts to gain access to the home-computer were unplanned.

## Conclusions

Effective parental support of children's home-computing has been related to two main factors: parental beliefs and attitudes, and the school's willingness for cooperation with the families. Research demonstrated parents' global positive expectations from the use of computers for their disabled children, pinpointing quantitative differences between fathers' and mothers' attitudes and beliefs. Overall, fathers expressed higher expectations than mothers, related to both their children's present and future needs. In-depth study is needed to further understand the complex systemic aspects of processes affecting home-computing, and an investigation of fathers' roles deserves special attention. Although research has emphasized their importance in fostering the growth and adjustment of their children, fathers have been found to accept a role of mother's-helper, demonstrating a less unique "male" role in families of disabled children. The increased enthusiasm from computers implies new possibilities for the father's role; however, Naisbitt's (1984) cautionary remarks, that increased expectations may reflect an attempt to reduce personal responsibilities, must be carefully considered.

Individual differences between families with regard to computer experiences, attitudes, and expectations emphasized the need for an individualistic approach to support planning. Most often, fathers wanted to be more involved in their children's home-computing than did mothers, yet in several families, this situation was reversed: These fathers expressed their alienation from technology, while the mothers were more cooperative and helpful. In addition, a gap was evident between beliefs and performance. Most parents expressed positive expectations from the computer impact, yet only several parents were either able or ready to devote time and efforts toward achieving the expected results. Intervention planning must attend to these individual differences.

Home-school interrelations may also affect the home-computing of disabled children, and research has shown that these contacts have been infrequent and unplanned, with limited effectiveness in using computers to bridge home and school performance. The ability to assess all of the parameters related to the development of a model for effective parental support of their children's home-computing, calls for a detailed study of the present, unplanned introduction and integration of computers into homes.

# 10

# Bringing the Computer Home

The growth of interest in developing a model for effective parental support in the home-computing of disabled children calls for an investigation of the introduction and integration of computers into homes. In order to study the ecological aspects of technology diffusion as related to the locations and usages of computers within the home environment of mildly disabled children, and parental support for the children's home-computing, an additional survey was conducted at Tel-Aviv University (Margalit, Rochberg, & Greenberg, 1988). The survey pinpointed three main aspects:

1 Diffusion of innovations.
2 Computer usages in these homes.
3 Parental characteristics as technology users.

Families who already owned computers participated in the second survey and were analyzed as detailed case studies: 36 families were interviewed in their homes and 24 families at Tel-Aviv University. No significant differences were found between the two groups of parents with regard to socio-economic variables or home-computing practices. In 39 of the families surveyed, the disabled child had been diagnosed with learning disabilities, and in 21 families, the disabled child had been diagnosed with mild mental retardation. The parents reported that their disabled children had been assessed by a school psychologist as a result of their learning difficulties and/or delayed development. The sample included 43 boys and 17 girls. All of the children were elementary school students, with an age range of 5 to 15 years (5-8 years = 21 children; 9-12 years = 26 children; and 13-15 years = 13 children). All of the families were intact families, with the exception of two single-parent families headed by mothers, in which the mothers and the children reported frequent contacts with the fathers.

## The diffusion of innovations

The study of the ecological environment among families with home-computers should encompass the factors affecting the decision making process for introducing computers into the homes of disabled children. In most families included in the Tel-Aviv University survey, the computer was relatively new at the time of the survey: 20 families (33.3%) had purchased the computer less than one year earlier; 28 (46.7%) families had bought the computer one to three years earlier, and only 12 families (20.0%) had made the computer purchase over four years earlier.

The study of the process of innovation diffusion among the homes of disabled children may clarify the different aspects of the decision making involved in buying a computer (Rogers, 1985). Technology innovations are diffused when they are spread out or become transmitted to others especially by contact. Diffusion comprises a special type of communication process. The main elements in the diffusion of new technologies are: an innovation (i.e., computer usage) that is communicated through certain channels (e.g., mass media or social networks), over time, among the members of a social system (i.e., families of disabled children). The spread of innovative new ideas involves some degree of uncertainty. The rate of the innovation's adoption and its style of usage are determined by the characteristics of the innovation, as perceived by the attitudes and expectations among members of the social system (i.e., the family members), as well as the characteristics of those families.

A communication channel constitutes the means by which messages are transmitted from one individual to another. The information regarding an innovation may be reached either through mass media channels or interpersonal networks. Rogers' (1985) study investigated the channels of communication used by families in order to obtain information on computers, regarding the manner in which parents realized that they required a computer and reached a decision regarding the selection of the particular computer that they eventually purchased. Rogers considered the mass media channels to be most effective in providing only general knowledge regarding the value of the innovations.

Interpersonal channels were regarded as more effective in forming and changing specific attitudes toward a new idea, which in turn influenced the decision to adopt or reject new ideas. Rogers (1985) reported that computers in the homes of nondisabled children were primarily diffused through close interpersonal peer networks and less through the mass-media. In the Tel-Aviv University survey, parents also reported that interpersonal networks (e.g., mostly social and vocational contacts who were knowledgeable about the technology) affected the decision making. However, the initial information about computers' advantages for disabled children also reached some families through mass-media channels: 8 families (13.3%) reported reading in a newspaper about computer usages for mentally retarded individuals, 20 (33.3%) attended a lecture about technology applications for disabled children, and 3 families (5.0%) reported viewing a television program demonstrating the computers' communicative role for cerebral palsied individuals.

The entrance of the computer into the home was not a completely novel experience for most disabled children. They had already gained some prior experience with computers either at school or at a special social club before acquiring a computer at home. The spread of the innovation -- the computer -- was not planned or guided. Most parents reported that the idea was introduced to them through mass-media channels or social networks. It remains a source of disappointment that the school was not the initiator of innovation diffusion. However, it should be mentioned that several parents' organizations initiated workshops for parents of disabled children to introduce the new technology usages.

## Decision making: Purchase

Some parents purchased their computers in order "to introduce modernity" into their homes, first consulting shop dealers and successful owners. Another important consideration in the decision making was the type of machine available at their children's schools. However, schools did not initiate consultation with regard to the child's particular needs that could be addressed by the computer, or with respect to the actual hardware and software available at the child's school. Parents in several families did not even contact the school in order to acquire the needed information, but rather asked the disabled child to provide them with the name of the machine that he/she used at school.

Four families (6.0%) expressed regret with regard to the computers they had selected. One family visited several shops and purchased a computer that was new and relatively rare among homes in Israel, and for which almost no educational software in Hebrew and only a few games were available. Another family complained bitterly that they had bought their computer according to their child's report of what the school was using, and soon afterwards the child moved to a special junior-high school that used a different type of machine. The support this family expected to receive from the new school in advising them in the use of educational software seemed unobtainable, as teachers at the new school used software that was not available for their machine. The surprising finding was that the parents did not contact the school in the first place. They assumed that the school could help them, but never actually asked for consultation with regard to the type of machine and software needed by their child.

Additional families complained that they did not know who to consult, and they expressed the feeling that their decision regarding the computer's purchase was not based on professional knowledge, but rather on a brief survey of machines owned by their friends or their children's friends. Only in five homes (8.3%) had a professional (e.g., pediatric neurologist, psychologist, school teacher) suggested the computer in order to assist and support the disabled children and as a partial answer to their difficulties.

With respect to the family member who made the decisions regarding the computer purchase, it was found that in more than half of the homes (33 homes - 55.0%), the fathers realized the family's needs and decided which computer to buy, and in 18 families (30.0%) both parents shared the decision. A nondisabled sibling was the decision maker in five families (e.g., as a present for a birthday or a Bar-Mitzvah), and the disabled children made all of the inquiries and participated actively in the decision making only in two homes.

Although the mothers in most families were reported to fully support the decision to buy the computer, they generally did not initiate the decision making. Only among three families, two of which were single-parent families, did mothers make the decisions about buying the computers. It can be concluded that fathers have a major role in introducing computers into the home, either by themselves or together with the mothers. However, in most families surveyed, the decision was supported by all the family members.

## Computer usages in the home

Typical users of computers at home as well as in the office usually experience a brief period characterized by a high level of frustration and anxiety. During this stressful period, users need help, support, and sometimes modeling in effective usages of the computer. If this assistance is not available, or is provided by a technology professional who is not aware and accepting of the difficulties and anxiety experienced by novice users, an aversion to the new instrument may develop. Awareness of this dynamic has significance for the understanding not only of the disabled child's reluctance to use the new technology, but also of the parents' empowering role in supporting their children's efforts.

Disabled children with learning difficulties require more extensive amounts of time and greater assistance in developing any new skill. Parents may effectively support the development of these skills only if they themselves overcome the initial stage of frustration and insecurity. In homes where parents expressed their ignorance and reluctance toward computers, the uses of computers were found to be minimal. On the other hand, in homes where parents used word-processors or any other computer usages extensively for their own work, acknowledging its benefits, more success was evident in helping the children to use the computers. In time, depending on the home environment, novice users either did or did not gain satisfaction from microcomputers, but those who became satisfied began to actively promote computers to others. Only in homes where parents regarded computer literacy not as a complicated, difficult skill, but rather as a challenge worthy of energy investment, could parents provide meaningful support for their disabled children.

An additional important aspect was the machine's reliability. Only expert users with technological training viewed mechanical difficulties as a challenge. Most users wanted any machine to perform smoothly, and in cases where the hardware or the software demonstrated operating difficulties, most parents and children decreased their home-computing time, experiencing feelings of anger and helplessness.

Following the decision to introduce a computer into the home environment, the following two major aspects of the home-computer's usage must be considered:

1 The physical placement or location of the computer hardware.
2 The software uses among the various family members.

## Location

Ergonomics or human engineering has become an important consideration in planning computer work environments that promote greater work efficiency, productivity, and comfort (Fernberg, 1985; Gross & Chapnik, 1987). Research on the design of the computer workplace has largely focused on employees in their worksetting. Little research attention has been devoted to the location and design of the computer environment in the home (Katz, 1988), and particularly as it relates to exceptional children's home-computing.

The location of the computer and the design of the computer workstation is profoundly affected not only by the characteristics of the tasks performed on the computer at home, but also by critical dynamic factors in the family system. The location has a powerful continuous impact on central aspects within the dynamic familial system, such as the family's patterns of interaction, the individual's right for privacy, inter-member territoriality struggles, and the status and power of the family members. Special environmental conditions are needed in order to enable computer users to function optimally, and individuals function best with microcomputing in their homes only when certain socio-psychological needs are met. The more time one spends on a computer, the greater one's need for adequate space conditions, although this rule of thumb is heavily influenced by the demands of the particular tasks and by the users' characteristics. Disabled children with specific learning difficulties, such as attention deficits and a low frustration tolerance due to continuous difficulties and failures, call for special consideration and planning.

## Decision making: Placement

The decision regarding the placement of the computers in the homes of these families was usually made after the computer's purchase. Most parents reported that during the first stage of discussing the computer purchase, they reached the decision to buy a computer but did not invest effort in planning its location in the home, or if so, they assumed that the computer would simply be placed in an available space. Only at a later stage did parents realize the large impact of the computer's location on its users.

> *Mr. B., the father of a learning disabled child, typified the families' decision making processes when he described his family's computer purchase and placement: "The decision of which machine to buy was a very difficult one. All our energy was invested in doing the right thing. When at last we had all the boxes at home, we found that we didn't know where to put the computer. We just hadn't thought about appropriate pieces of furniture. Here the kids were, all excited about bringing the new computer home, and in the end, we had to leave the computer in the box until we were able to find somewhere to put it."*

Available space and special custom-made computer furniture were often related to the families' economic situation and income. In addition, the individual family members' physical or socio-psychological needs were rarely considered. Computers were usually placed wherever a convenient space was found, with little consideration paid to the users' workplace needs, such as physical comfort, lighting, or noise. Katz (1988), in a study of home-computing locations, found that as many families chose a shared family area (41%) as those who chose an individual, private space (43%). Only three families had set up what they called a "computer room," a separate room for the computer.

The present survey, similarly to Katz's (1988) findings for the homes of nondisabled children, demonstrated that computers may be found in almost any room in the house, from the kitchen to the corridor to the bedroom. However, most locations could be categorized as either private space or common family space, and as either adult areas or child areas. As can be seen on Figure 10.1, in 27 families (45.1%) the computer was located in a common family space. Of these families, the living room was the computer's location in 8 homes (13.3%), and in the remaining 19 homes (31.7%), it was placed in one of various family spaces such as work room, corridor, or game room. Only one family reported having a special computer room.

About half of the families viewed the children as the main users and placed the computer in the children's rooms in 31 homes (51.7%). Of these homes, the computer was located in the disabled child's room in 14 homes (23.3%), and in the sibling's room in the remaining 17 families (28.3%). In five

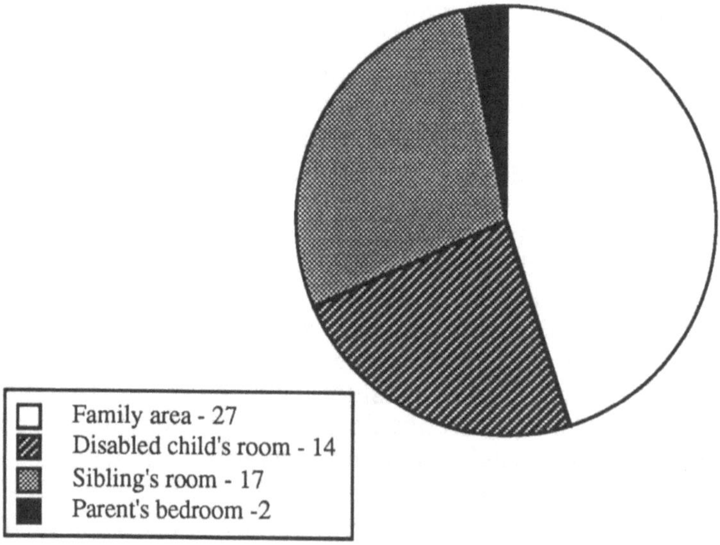


Figure 10.1. Placement of the home-computer

families, the computer had been a Bar-Mitzvah present to the oldest sibling, and was placed in his/her room, acknowledging that particular child's ownership, but maintaining availability to other family members. The computer was placed in the parents' bedroom only in two families (3.3%), and one of these machines was later transferred to the living room, where it was more easily accessible to the children.

The decision regarding the selection of the room in which to place the computer depended on several additional factors related to developmental and interpersonal needs among family members. Family usage of the computer was affected by the children's need for privacy, which varies with the stages in the life cycle. A clear difference exists between the definitions of younger and adolescent children's privacy or territory needs. Teenagers seek privacy, and their territorial boundaries are well defined. When the computer was located in an adolescent child's bedroom, other members of the family, especially younger siblings, were less able to use the machine. As mentioned above, some computers were bought as gifts for the adolescent siblings, further emphasizing their ownership of the machine.

Sibling rivalry also occurred among younger children, with the older of the two usually victorious. Younger children's territorial boundaries become more defined only as they get older; thus, placing a computer in their room has less impact on the other family members. Younger children and sometimes disabled children often felt even more comfortable being surrounded by other members of the family and also more frequently needed supervision while using the machine.

In summary, the computer in most homes was placed in a space shared by all the family members (or especially by the children), and which was easily accessible to all of the children. Only in 21 homes (35.0%) was the computer placed in a private space (i.e., child's or parent's room): either in the disabled child's room, in another sibling's room (usually an older one), or, rarely, in the parents' bedroom. The placement of the computer in the disabled child's room was related not to the severity of his or her difficulties, but rather to the goals of the computer purchase.

## Software usages by various family members

The entrance of recent technologies into the home may be expected to affect the family environment and life style. Family system dynamics may adjust to the presence of computers, just as families have already adapted their life style to telephones, televisions, and other recent technology. The noticeable impact of these "older" technologies on leisure activities and social interrelations suggests that computers may also be expected to affect family interactional patterns. However, it appears that family dynamics will continue to be in control of what computers will and will not do. Like other new arrivals, the computer will only be one more occasion for the prevailing family patterns to be both reasserted and modified (Hunt, 1985). Computers establish either competitive or cooperative situations in the family, creating opportunities for modeling effective learning, problem solving, and work patterns. The exploration of effective software use among families with disabled children should first address the critical needs of each of the family members.

Wright and Church (1986) focused interest on the differences between computer usages in the home and classroom. In the classroom, where the computer must be shared, it can be considered a scarce resource. At home, being available almost all of the time, the computer may be viewed as a free resource. For example, one parental volunteer (Wright & Church, 1986) reported that his daughter could accomplish far more than was revealed only by her work on the computer in the classroom. He reported that at home, his daughter could be helped to use the program for an initial period of time, and sufficient time then remained for her to continue using the program independently, as she wished. At school her computer time was limited, and when she experimented with the program's usages, there were already other students waiting for their turns.

The current Tel-Aviv survey of families with disabled children corroborated an interesting finding reported by Dede and Gottlieb (1984) in their study of home-computing among 100 families with nondisabled children. Users tended to underestimate the amount of time that they spent with the computer, complaining of a feeling that "time runs more quickly" when they are working on the computer, and wishing for more computer time. Some even called the computer a "time eater," feeling that they usually spent more time with the computer than they originally intended. In our study, parents reported that even hyperactive children with concentration difficulties, who usually found it difficult to maintain any activity for more than a few minutes, tended to work for longer periods on the computer.

The most common software usages for home-computers among children and adults were found to be:

1 Computer games.
2 Parental work usages.
3 Children's homework and word processing.

## Computer games

Playing computer games was usually found to be the children's primary computer activity, and a widespread acceptance and support of game playing was demonstrated by the parents of disabled and nondisabled children alike. Only seven families with disabled children reported that none of the family members played computer games during the survey period. In most homes, the children constituted the primary game players and the parents (mostly fathers) continuously provided the family with new games and sometimes participated in the activity. An older nondisabled sibling was often found to play the role of tutor and computer game "expert" or to share this role with the father. The disabled children's functioning was variable: In most homes they required intensive help and guidance in their initial interactions with the new technology, and some needed continuous adult support. However, 35 (58.3%) disabled children (mostly learning disabled males) achieved independent and fluent game abilities of which they were very proud.

An interesting phenomenon was remarked upon in many homes, where the fathers rather proudly stated that their children, even the disabled ones, had developed skilled performance in playing games and were even better players than the fathers themselves. This situation may constitute a rare occasion when even very young or disabled children can develop a sense of excellent performance. For handicapped children, who most frequently experience a sense of frustration and failure, and who feel they often disappoint their parents, the importance of an ability to win at computer games against a parental opponent cannot be underestimated. Both the parent and the disabled child thus enjoy a sense of pride and excitement which make a strong contribution to their self-esteem and interrelations.

Similarly to the impact attributed to video games (Mitchell, 1985), computer games were highlighted in the current survey as responsible for bringing families together for common recreational interactions and shared play, more than any other computer activity. However, in general, the excitement and the amount of time allotted to game play in the family decreased several months after the games entered the home. Only in homes where the parents were actively engaged in continuously providing new games, was the interest level maintained. Two additional aspects of computer game playing were raised by several families:

1 Several games, even after the initial excitement had decreased, remained a center of family interest. Except for the traditional games such as chess, it was rather difficult to predict which games would survive over time.
2 Despite strong sex differences in participation interest and skill level, the game activity provided many female members of the family (both child and adult) with an opportunity to engage and succeed in an activity which they considered male dominated and male oriented.

For playing games, the placement of the computer held specific importance. The optimal location of the computer for game playing was in a common space where several family members had free access, in order to play jointly, compare achievements, encourage and advise the novice player, and treat the games as shared family leisure activities.

## Parents' work-related uses

Parental work-related computer usages (e.g., word processing, business software) predominated among 36.7% of the families in the Tel-Aviv University survey (i.e. 22 homes), as compared to 25% in Katz's (1988) study of families without disabled children. The use of the computer for these parents took precedence over their children's, and in these homes, the computers were usually located in the family room or in two cases, in the parents' bedroom. These parents expressed a strong need for a quiet space in which to work on the computer for long periods without interference. Heavier restrictions were placed on the computer's use in these families; for example, in one home only the father used the computer, and the children were not allowed to operate it. In several other homes where the computer was considered a work tool, the disabled child was not permitted to use it without adult supervision.

## Children's homework and word processing

Only 14 parents (23.3%) in the Tel-Aviv University survey reported that their children used academic software, mostly drill-and-practice, and in only five homes the children used a word processor occasionally. As Papert (1980) has pointed out, word processing consists of an adult, professional use of the computer which has become available to children. This may be the reason why many parents felt more inclined to assist in their children's word processing than in other activities. Those parents who used word processing programs regularly and enthusiastically themselves were more likely to take on the role of teacher to their children, thereby modeling the role of active learner (Bruner, 1985). This phenomenon emphasized an additional aspect of child-parent interactions that will be considered below: the extent to which the parent felt relaxed with the computer.

As continual contact between school and home was absent, parents were rarely aware of the types of software in use in their children's schools. In addition, mothers and fathers frequently complained that their children were bored by the academic software that they brought home from school, and that they attempted to avoid academic training. These parents' disappointment, following their high expectations that their children would demonstrate great motivation to practice learning in subjects that comprised areas of difficulty, was the subject of frustration and annoyance. However, it should be remembered that in almost all families, computer activity was regarded as complementary rather than compulsory, and as an inadequate substitute for the mandatory homework assigned in difficult subjects. The parents valued computer activity as less important than homework and remedial learning, and rules were often made in the family, placing computer work as last priority, following all of the children's other learning activities.

## Computer not in use

Several of the computers in the families surveyed were rarely used or were not used at all. In two families, the computers had been sent out for repairs, and the parents' lack of ability to specify any approximate date for the computers' return expressed the parents' loss of interest. In two other homes, none of the family members operated the computer any longer, emphasizing the parents' reluctance and disinterest in the computer, as well as their inability to assist their children in its use. When the survey interviewers expressed acceptance of the parental attitude and inquired regarding the parents' reasons for purchasing their computers, several parents explained:

> *Mr. V.: "I saw my children's friends and their enthusiasm for their home-computers, and I just assumed that my children would also be really active in using the computer. My kids got really excited about the idea, and the truth is that they just pressured me into making the purchase. I believed they would use it."*

> *Mrs. K.: "At first, all of my kids quarreled for computer time and were very interested, but their interest sure faded quickly. Now they are all excited about the new electronic organ."*

The interviewers' impression was that these family members viewed the computer as a new toy and not as a tool. As a new toy, when the novice effect faded, the computer no longer held its attraction. In addition, due to the fact that the computer's advantages as a useful tool were not firmly established in the family, after some time a new and more exciting toy was adopted.

## Parental characteristics as technology users

In the study of computer usage at home, consideration should be given to parental characteristics which may affect critical aspects in the adoption of the technology, and parental ability to provide assistance and support. Various parental characteristics affect home-computing: parents' role overload; their availability and involvement in their children's learning in general, and learning with computers in particular; parental familiarity and experience with computers and relevant software; and the extent to which the parents feel comfortable with and are attracted to the microcomputer.

For many of the interviewed parents, technology was not of personal interest to them and left them feeling uninvolved or even anxious and uneasy. Many of these parents described their purchase of the computer as a:

1 Reaction to the pressure of their children;
2 Gesture signifying help-giving to their children;
3 Compensation for either disabilities or overinvolvement with the disabled child;
4 Expression of interest in modernity (i.e., "*bringing the 21st century home*").

Although they revealed increased expectations from the computer's potential impact on their children's difficulties, parents often expressed the conviction that their involvement in their children's home-computing ended with the purchase of the computer. In those homes where parents felt alienated from the computers, the computer's range of usage and the amount of time spent working with it were found to decrease sharply after the initial overall excitement.

### Computer literacy stages

Another aspect in the dynamics of parental attitudes, which should also be considered within the planning of an intervention model, is related to the expected stages reported by Hunt (1985) for becoming a computer user. Not only the parents, but each one of the family members, may be described as functioning at one of the following stages:

1 *Fearful user*: The new user may feel overwhelmed by fear, anxiety, and expectations for an unpleasant experience.
2 *Entranced user*: The new user may feel fascination with the mystery and the power of the machine, including an acceptance of expected difficulties, yet also a willingness to try and experience new computer applications.
3 *Beginner*: The new user begins learning to use the computer, following instructions meticulously or even in a rigid manner, feeling certain that everyone knows more than he or she does.
4 *Experienced users*: In this stage the user is ready to try new, additional options for familiar programs, and he or she even attempts to take shortcuts in skilled procedures, sometimes to the point of carelessness and of ignoring procedures necessary for successful operation.
5 *Frustrated realist*: The experienced and overexcited user may feel disillusion, discovering that the computer cannot do everything that the user originally imagined would be possible. He or she may develop an awareness of the cost of their home-computing in terms of time investment and personal tension.
6 *Sophisticated user*: The experienced users and realists discover and accept the computer's possibilities and limitations as a tool.

Each family member can be expected to fall at a somewhat different step in this progression of fluency, and the parents' literacy stage may affect their ability to support their disabled child's progression toward fuller computer literacy. In a study attempting to empower parents' capability to support their children's home-computing, several groups of parents began learning basic computer skills (Dik, 1984). The results of the study demonstrated that, as the parents strengthened their skills in the area of computer literacy, they became empowered to enter into the teaching and learning process, and to be more effective in supporting their children's computer work.

## Family member computer interactions

Parent-child computer interactions prior to any attempt to carry out an experimental intervention, were categorized into household rules reflecting parental support, using Wolins' (1988) conceptualization. Parents constructed household rules relating to the home-computing, such as the amount of time that a child may spend working/playing with the computer, or rules granting equal access or priority to competing siblings. These rules reflected family dynamics (i.e., which family members possessed greater power and resources) as well as parental attitudes toward the computer (i.e., as an educational tool or as a toy for entertainment). These household rules included some of the following examples found among the parents interviewed:

1 *No computer usage is allowed when the family needs the room for social interactions (e.g., entertaining guests, watching TV).*
2 *The disabled child comes first.*
3 *Parents' work has priority over children's usages.*
4 *The older sibling gets more time.*
5 *School-related activities such as homework receive priority, and computer usages (even academically related ones) are secondary.*
6 *Within computer activities, word processing comes first and games afterwards.*
7 *Younger or disabled children cannot use the computer unless the father is present.*

At times, the prevailing rules betrayed attitudes which were contradictory to those that were stated directly by parents. Parents may have claimed, for example that the computer had been purchased for the children, but actually the father's work was found to have priority. In many families, the children's computer activity was considered as important for their education and growth, even more important than school, yet the children were allowed to use computers only after completing their homework.

Parents' support for their children's home-computing was demonstrated in several ways. Parents expressed verbal support through praise, encouragement, and positive reinforcement. The handicapped child was often reported to use the computer in the presence of other family members who cheered him/her on, and the child even demonstrated newly acquired skills to grandparents and occasionally to guests. Parents also provided physical support in terms of sitting down with the child at the computer. Usually, fathers attempted to provide assistance to the disabled child. In many homes computer-related interactions exemplified the most intensive area of involvement between fathers and their disabled children, whereas mothers were found to be more active in all of the other needed areas.

*Mrs. L.: Hopes for husband and son*

*Mrs. L., a mother of a 7-year-old mentally retarded boy, said that their computer had been purchased in order to develop a common interest between her husband and disabled son. Mr. L. personally found computer usage very appealing. Mrs. L. expressed her wish that her husband would share his attraction to technology with their son, and that the computer would thus serve as a bridge between father and son, who shared little in common. It should be noted that Mr. L. was present during the entire interview, but he kept his involvement to a minimum, only nodding in supportive acceptance of Mrs. L.'s words.*

*Mrs. T.: A reluctant professional programmer*

*Mrs. T., a mother of a 9-year-old boy with an attention deficit disorder, works as a professional computer programmer and enjoys her job. However, she consistently failed to help her son with his attempts to use their home-computer, and she expressed great reluctance to getting involved in her son's activities with regard to home-computing. Despite her greater expertise and knowledge, Mrs. T. encouraged and supported her husband's dominant role in supporting his son's experimentations with the computer.*

Children very rarely played the role of teachers for their parents, although most of the children had learned to use computers independently in school. Only a few parents thought about asking their children for guidance and help. Sometimes parents remarked that their children were ready and willing to show the software to anybody interested, yet the parents themselves simply never asked for assistance.

*Mr. and Mrs. Y. were reluctant to use technology, distancing themselves from the computer activity. Their younger nondisabled son accepted a dominating role in helping his older disabled sibling. The parents in this family expressed pride in their young child's expertise.*

The interrelations between siblings constitute another aspect of the family system that should be considered. Not only did parents demonstrate or guide children's learning on the computer, but siblings did as well, usually in game playing and less commonly in school-related subjects. Sibling support was most common during game playing, especially when the software (e.g., an adventure game) demanded the participation of an opponent. Sibling support was less common during computer use for school-related tasks such as word processing. In several families, one of the children became the major user of the home-computer, usually the brighter male, and other siblings who may have needed it more, such as those with learning difficulties, had to struggle and required parental support in order to acquire frequent access to the computer.

Clear sex role differences were noted during the interviews. Mothers in most families used the computer less often than the fathers, mostly for word processing, and treated it as a tool. Several mothers expressed their reluctance and even alienation from the computer, while others complained that "they don't get to the computer till late at night," blaming their work overload at home, and the caring duties related to the disabled child. Fathers, on the other hand, expressed their enjoyment from the new "toy," reporting their varied uses such as game-playing, programming, and work applications.

## Conclusions

The analysis shows that the location of the computer in the home and the design of the computer workplace created an impact on the home-microcomputing in families with disabled children. However, little consideration was paid to the physical comfort, lighting, noise, or other workplace needs of the user, resulting in poor interactions between the child and the microcomputer environment. Most families were not aware of the users' needs and family dynamics, and their decisions concerning the placement and usage of the microcomputer were usually made after the purchase.

Often the location was determined by the home conditions such as spatial or structural limitations or by the family member who had the most power in the family system. The ages and developmental stages of the children in the family also played a role in decisions related to the computer's introduction into the home. Young children often require supervision and feel more secure in using the computer when in the company of parents or older siblings. Placing the computer in a teenager's room emphasized a need for privacy and a tendency to protect territorial boundaries, whereas its location in a parentally controlled room affected the rest of the family's style of usage. The placement of the computer reflects family dynamics, influencing effective usages. Hunt (1985) even suggested that teaching computer skills to family members be used as a way to model and demonstrate effective communication principles with other family members, as the computer only does what you tell it to do, not what you think you have told it or want it to do (Hunt, 1985).

Several implications for a more effective microcomputer environment were revealed. An ecological approach should be used in the design of the microcomputer environment, in order to evaluate the changing needs of the family as it grows and to continuously assess the interactions between the users and their environment. An attempt should also be made to develop a functional workstation providing personal privacy and resulting in minimal distractions and increased productivity. The users' comfort and fulfilled needs may contribute to their well-being and control over their environment, resulting in increased productivity. The importance of appropriate skills should also be considered imperative for meaningful, beneficial computer interactions. The development and acquisition of computer skills constitutes a challenge for family members of all ages, and parents can play an active role in assisting their disabled children to meet this challenge.

The designing of activities for disabled children on home-computers calls for integrating computer usages into everyday contexts. One of the advantages of everyday learning consists of the fact that it usually takes place in the context of meaningful activities. For example, word processing and game playing were the frequent uses found in several studies. In order to support the children's activities, parents should, for instance, attempt to develop their own word processing skills, and to practice playing games with their children. In general, parents must devote some thought to integrating their own computer usages at home and work, including occupational and leisure activities. Parental attention directed toward their own attitudes regarding the use and potential of technology is essential in order to define goals for their children's use. Thinking about the computer as a tool calls for enhancing the computer activities that are already often performed without computers. Parents can reflect upon the ways they learn new things -- reading a book, writing notes, working cooperatively with a friend -- thus serving as a model for learning something new of an intellectual nature.

Parents can be effective agents for educating their children. They can foster incidental learning opportunities in the home context. They can model successful learning procedures, structure situations for direct teaching at the computer, and provide children with verbal and physical support during their computing experiments. Descriptions of strategies to empower parents in their support of the children's home-computing will be detailed in Chapter 11.

# 11

# Parental Support of Children's Home-Computing

In an attempt to develop an effective model of empowering parents in their involvement and support of their children's home-computing, ecological considerations and cognitive and emotional variables affecting the children's home-computing will be identified and examined. Special attention will be directed toward aspects related to the effectiveness of different teaching methods for engaging children in various tasks and situations. Two types of strategies, essential in order to develop an effective model for parents' intervention, will be detailed:

1. Training parents to support their children's successful experience with computers and to develop and reinforce home-school involvement.
2. Training parents to tutor and teach their children in their home-computing.

The latter role, of parents as teachers, places greater demands and is characterized more by specific definitions of time and place than the former role of parent as a supporter of the processes. In both roles the nature of the parent-child interaction plays a central part and will be discussed. An individualistic and dynamic approach to intervention in this area will be presented. The model can be considered individualistic in the sense that it enables adaptation to children's specific needs and to parents' available personal resources. The proposed approach may be described as dynamic as a result of its openness to changes that reflect periodic transitions. Such transitions may occur from periods of familial stress and overload either at home or at work, which are either related or unrelated to the specific difficulties of the disabled child, to periods when the parents want and feel able to devote more time and energy to meeting their children's needs, and to taking an active role in changing their children's present situation.

## Support of home-computing

Parental support of disabled children's home-computing can be divided into (a) planned support of the children's performance, with an emphasis on home-school interrelations, and (b) a global, supportive family climate with an emphasis on a wide range of computing activities for the family members.

## Planned support

The goal of the planned support strategy focuses on reinforcing the home-school interrelations in order to ensure continuity between school experience and the child's experiences at home, aiming to:

1 Increase the impact of the educational curriculum on the children's development through professionalized parental roles;
2 Assist parents to become more efficiently involved in their children's development, without changing parents' primary parental role; and
3 Develop a bridge between school and home micro-computing activity, through parents' training in measures which support and reinforce their children's performance.

The present intervention plan was guided by the realization that parents wish to know more about their children's abilities and difficulties, to extend the impact of educational processes through their support in the home, and to participate in decision making and advocacy activities (Allen & Stefanowski-Hudd, 1987). The advantages of the proposed type of intervention programs lie in the fact that they attempt to avoid creating additional obligations for the already overloaded parents, while accentuating the provision of support and reinforcement to parents' involvement in their children's computing.

## Parent-child interactions

In a recent study, Mahoney and Powel (1988) identified characteristics of parent-child interrelations that were considered to be closely related to children's development. These researchers emphasized the importance of parenting style, as defined by characteristics such as sensitivity to children's needs, achievement orientation, warmth of interrelations, responsiveness to children's communications, and enjoyment. Among parents of handicapped children, Mahoney and Powel (1988) considered two aspects of parental interaction style to be relatively ineffective in promoting children's development: directiveness and unresponsiveness. For example, the developmental level of mentally retarded children (Mahoney, Finger & Powel, 1985) was found to be related to three dimensions of maternal behavioral style:

1 Child orientation.
2 Quantity of stimulation.
3 Control.

The children with the highest developmental scores had mothers whose interactive style was characterized by a high degree of child orientation and responsiveness, and a low degree of control, combined with an increased amount of stimulation in the home environment. In another study, Mahoney (1988) found that children who were the least communicative had mothers who tended to be unresponsive to children's communication. Observations revealed that in mother-child interactions these mothers focused their communication on directing children to attend to the mothers' own topics of conversation.

The active attempts by parents to obtain their children's optimal levels of behavior have been described as a strategy that frequently leads to high levels of directiveness and intrusiveness and less responsiveness to the child's efforts. Such activity may be regarded as a natural consequence among families with disabled children, who manifest frustrating behaviors such as passivity, and who generally constitute problematic social partners for communication with their parents. An interactional pattern emerges, where the handicapped child's presence in the family, characterized by irritating inactivity, stimulates the parents, who respond by trying to fill up the communicational emptiness through overactivity. At the same time, disabled children, realizing their small effect on the nonresponsive and overactive parent, tend gradually to develop behavioral patterns of learned helplessness, increased passivity, and a diminished contingency awareness.

The results from several intervention studies (Mash & Terdal, 1973; Seitz & Hoekenga, 1974) have indicated that more normalized styles of interaction may be within both the child's and the mother's repertoires of behavior, yet the results revealed that, due to an apparent interactive breakdown, these desired behaviors fail to occur. If parents can learn which aspects of their disabled child's behavior tend to elicit high frequencies of directive parental behavior and why, they may also be able to learn how to decrease the frequencies of these directive, unresponsive interaction patterns and how to increase their own communicative patterns. Lack of parental attention to their own emotional and communicative responses to their children's behavior may result in a communication breakdown in the parent-child interaction.

An additional aspect of parent-child interactions lies in the fact that parents frequently bring to the interactions with their disabled children a negative set of expectancies. The achievement levels of disabled children are often lower than those of their peer group, but even so more efforts are needed in order to reach these lower achievement levels. The children's sensitivity to verbal and nonverbal parental behavior, which expresses their expectations and beliefs regarding the children's capacities, must play an important part in the parents' training.

Research (Block, 1983) has further suggested that mothers and fathers interact differently with their children: Fathers, for example, tend to be more didactic than mothers in their interactions. Fathers' nonverbal behavior was studied through investigating father-son interactions during their work on a computer, and fathers' body language and smiling behavior was found to have a significant impact on their son's cognitive development (Tremblay, Larivee & Gregoire, 1985).

The various studies presented here share important

implications for the integration of the computer into the home of the disabled child. The findings regarding the effect of parental nonverbal, communicative, and emotional tendencies when confronted by their handicapped children's behavior constitutes striking evidence that serious thought, attention, and awareness should be devoted by these parents to their interactions with their children concerning the computer. Disabled children require increased supervision and guidance, not only in the cognitive realm, but also in dealing with the emotional aspect of the computer's entrance into the family, with all of its ramifications for the family's lifestyle.

## Shared interests

The parents' role does not begin and end with the purchase of the home-computer. In order to foster their children's technology usage, parents must discover how and when computers become interesting for themselves. The identification of meaningful activities for both parent and child may significantly foster parental support of children's computing through unique parent-child interactions characterized by a sense of togetherness and mutual concern and interest. These activities will not contribute to consistent, long-term, and productive maternal and paternal supportive involvement unless they consist not only of a direct reply to the disabled child's specific needs, but also rest within the range of parental interests. Heard and Lake (1986) found that individuals have a natural propensity to develop interpersonal interactions and companionship with those persons who have a similar commitment to sharing one or more interests. This tendency serves the function of providing both shared awareness and understanding of an interest, and the recognition of an area of personal competence. The goal of such companionable interaction can be reached during the sharing of new information and skills associated with an interest. Through both verbal and non-verbal language during the sharing of such knowledge or ability, each participant conveys the feelings, thoughts, and wishes each has about the behavior of the other.

Forming close relations with one's disabled child frequently constitutes a difficult task for parents, arousing many feelings associated with the parents' acceptance of the differences between their disabled child and his or her nondisabled peers. Fathers often develop companionable interrelations with their nonhandicapped children; however, they encounter difficulty becoming involved in interactions that revolve around a shared interest with their disabled children. Despite tendencies in our society toward greater paternal involvement in childrearing and housekeeping, fathers of disabled children were usually found to treat such responsibilities as a uniquely maternal role, and whenever fathers were found to increase their involvement in these activities, they viewed their role as one of mother's helper (Gallagher, Beckman, & Cross, 1983). The integration of computers into the family environment may be utilized as a specific task which reflects a unique opportunity to assist fathers in becoming involved, through sharing an interest and developing companionable relations with their handicapped children. Fathers can be sensitized into realizing the emotive messages sent by these children when they are participating in a shared activity that represents a mutual father-child interest, and mothers may help encourage the process through showing appreciation of the father's contribution to his child's development in an area valued to the father. Demos (1988) demonstrated in his study that parents can even use various recent technological advances such as television, video cassette recorders, and computers to enhance their children's reading, writing, and problem solving skills through developing common interest areas.

Often parents think that they naturally support their children desired activity; however, through both verbal and nonverbal communication, parents express their actual beliefs and expectations regarding their children's performance, which may contradict their overtly stated attitudes. In addition, most parents seem unaware of the major beneficial impact that relations with their children's schools may have on the children's use of the home-computer. Consequently, an intervention program developed at Tel-Aviv University to assist parents in adaptatively supporting their children's computer performance comprised the following objectives: teaching parents to identify and support desirable computer activities of mutual interest to parent and child and with clear relevance to the child's specific needs; and training parents to acquire knowledge concerning the schools' goals and usages for hardware and software integration. In order to develop more focused parental support and reinforcement, and to extend the impact of school learning, the interventional program suggested several planned steps:

*Identification of meaningful areas for reinforcement.* Areas of significance for the children's development were pinpointed, in which the children showed the potential to succeed in their efforts, and which were related to parents' own areas of interest. Although some parents were already involved in home-computing, it should be emphasized that they often required prior training using the academic software employed in their children's schools, in order to develop a feeling of mastery and comfort with this activity. Yet, when home-computing actually interested parents, such training appeared less important than the parents' ability to model effective learning processes and coping strategies to the disabled child, regarding a new area of instruction or, more specifically, a new software program.

*Planning parental support of the children's performance as composed of two main parent-child interaction patterns: (a) interactions that respond to the children's activity, and (b) interactions initiating new activity.* In an attempt to reduce parental directiveness and unresponsiveness levels, the training was focused on parental listening and on identifying desired behavior. Although responsive behavior appears to have greater effectiveness in fostering development, the initiation of increased directive parental behavior often constitutes a more appropriate and necessary behavior in the face of disabled children's extreme passivity and learned helplessness. Parental self-awareness was directed toward (a) continuously evaluating and reevaluating the specific situational needs, (b) moving flexibly from one behavioral pattern to another, and (c) increasingly recognizing the natural parental tendency toward directive, unresponsive interactions whenever confronted by children's passivity.

*Planning verbal and nonverbal support, which reflect individual differences.* Some parental support is expressed verbally, for instance, congratulating children for their efforts, positively evaluating performance, or detailing various aspects of skill advancement. Support is also always expressed nonverbally, through facial expression, tone of voice, and body language such as a kiss, a smile, or attentive observation of the children's activity, demonstrating interest and involvement.

During the intervention meetings, parents were encouraged to list the types and number of reinforcement acts they provided to their children, and to share with other parents the descriptions of their supportive interactions. Parents were trained to support only meaningful achievements, yet not to wait passively for their occurrence, but rather to plan and create such opportunities for successful performance. In addition, parents were sensitized to their choice of words and to nonverbal interaction modes in their communication and were taught to develop a greater repertoire of alternative supportive expressions. In several families, the father was found to be the major supporter of the home-computing activities; therefore, mothers were encouraged to reinforce their husbands whenever they supported their disabled children's desired, pre-identified computer activity. Several fathers revealed emotional involvement with their children's home-computing, sometimes reporting the children's performance in a way that expressed a boost to the ego and an identification with the child's activity.

> *Mr. S. described his disabled child's computing in plural terms, saying "At the beginning, we found the software too difficult for us, but after intensive training we were able to increase our scores and speed."*

Meaningful involvement with the school's computing activities requires two interested partners. Surveys have demonstrated that without planned involvement, parents and teachers failed to discuss the school's computing activities. Although parents constantly expressed their wish during interviews to learn more about these activities, they did not initiate such interrelations. However, not only parents' training is needed to increase parental involvement in school-home-computing, but also teachers' training is essential for supporting parents in their efforts to extend the impact of the educational software at home. The supportive, complementary role of the teacher deserves further investigation.

## Supportive family climate

The disabled children's home-computing may be facilitated if several family members demonstrate their enthusiasm and their own wide range of computer usages. Clarifying with parents their aims in buying computers may reflect aspects of the family climate related to home-computing. Several parents reported during interviews that their computers had been purchased primarily to help the disabled child in the family with his/her academic difficulties. However, a more promising approach can be attempted through developing a computer-supported learning environment at home, in which the computer becomes a natural part of everyday life in the family, similarly to the television and the tape-recorder. In homes where the computer's single goal and use was to assist the disabled children, parents' interviews revealed that its usages had been gradually decreasing, and parents expressed their disappointment that the expected "miraculous" effects had not been demonstrated. In the reported survey, the most frequently reported computer usages among family members were:

1 As a tool (e.g., word processor, dictionary, data base program) to help family members in their work or homework.
2 As a leisure or recreational activity (e.g., playing different games, writing personal letters, or learning new computer languages) to be used during periods of free time.

It was also reported that in those homes where parents or older siblings consistently introduced new programs, continuing interest in computers and a willingness to experiment were demonstrated, thus modeling ways to learn new software programs. The disabled children in such families viewed computer performance as: an opportunity for a successful learning experience; a symbol of their belonging and participating in an area of common family interest; a means for establishing meaningful interrelations with other family members; and a tool for developing competency within an area valued by the family.

During the interviews, many parents raised questions regarding computer games. Parents expressed hesitation as to whether playing games should be treated as an acceptable activity for the disabled child. The important value of computer games for disabled children within the framework of effective problem solving, or as an interesting and independent leisure activity, has been described in Chapter 2. Appropriate parental support and reinforcement will not be spontaneous or sincere until parents clarify to themselves their own attitudes toward computer games, attempting to identify games' beneficial impact.

Two brief descriptions of interventions may portray the range of family environments that need be considered in planning parental support of their children's home-computing.

## Sammy S.: Insufficient computer access

In several of the surveyed families where the computer was in high demand, the disabled children did not receive enough computer time, creating a need for special parental rules regarding an order of preferences in the family.

> *Mr. S. reported that everyone in his family used the computer, and he was not aware that in this struggle for computer time, his 7-year-old dyslectic son (Sammy) was gradually using the computer less. During the interview the father realized the situation, and his subsequent inquiry revealed that whenever Sammy attempted to use the computer, he was gently pushed aside by his older brothers, who considered his performance and the type of software that he used at school as "childish" and "too simple," and who ridiculed Sammy's inability to play the more advanced computer games which required faster response times and increased skills.*
>
> *The father found that when Sammy tried to protest, one of the two brothers would frequently volunteer to "teach" Sammy to play "real" games, resulting in a typical scenario where Sammy passively watched the sibling play the game alone or with another peer. Sammy was helped to gain access to the computer through devising a set of family rules, including defined allocations of available computer time to every interested family member. In addition, the older brother was encouraged (via an incentive of increased computer time) to gradually teach Sammy to play the more complicated "adult games," and at the same time to express support of Sammy during his struggles and difficulties. Interestingly, after only a brief period of time, this elder brother became quite involved in Sammy's computer efforts and achievements, and was even able to regretfully express his initial feelings of*

*shame and alienation and his anxiety that his peers would ridicule Sammy's inabilities and lower performance levels.*

## Ron H.: An oppositional adolescent

In homes where the sole purpose of the computer purchase was to help the disabled child, who thus remained its sole user, the computer was quickly perceived as "just another" remedial activity. Consequently, many disabled children treated the computer as additional homework, attempting to avoid and delay this activity.

*Descriptions of the need for a range of flexible and individualized modes of parental support were provided by Mr. and Mrs. H. Their 14-year-old mildly retarded son, Ron, reached a phase in his development when he rejected his father's attempts to assist him in his home-computing. The teacher had given Mr. H. the software being used at school, anxious to encourage both parents to work with the program at home, as most of Ron's classmates had already mastered the software. Ron, who at that time revealed various expressions of his adolescence phase, also protested against the suggestion that he should work with his parents at home. Mr. and Mrs. H. then contacted the community involvement program at the local university and located a student to work as a "Big Brother" with Ron. Parental support was planned carefully, so as not to initiate the son's oppositional behavior tendencies. The following depicts the supportive strategies that were implemented by the parents, as well as the family's responses to the intervention:*

1. *The father consistently remarked on the increasing periods of training that Ron devoted to his computer activity.*
2. *Assuming that their son often eavesdropped to their conversations, the father and mother began to appreciatively talk about the efforts that Ron demonstrated in his computer activity, whenever it was obvious that Ron could be listening to them.*

*Although Ron pretended for a long time to ignore their conversations, one day they received confirmation of his attentive listening, when he suddenly corrected the mother angrily, saying that he had worked on the computer "for much longer than you said -- from four o'clock to five o'clock and not just from four until a quarter of five."*

3 *When Ron reported on his achievements, and even when his teacher at school praised Ron on his improved performance, each parent congratulated him, asking for his permission to tell his grandmother the good news. Eventually Ron even suggested that he would show off, and during his grandmother's next visit he insisted on operating the computer independently, while everybody expressed their excitement.*

4 *When Ron was working on the computer, Mr. H. smiled at him without saying anything or patted him on the back, and Mrs. H. sometimes even "shushed" Ron's younger nondisabled sister, instructing her to play quietly with her girlfriends and not to interfere with Ron's computer activity.*

5 *Mr. and Mrs. H. attempted to perform at least two supportive activities each day, and to report them to one another at the end of each day. They remarked that at first they felt that they did not like the artificial aspects of the support planning; however, soon they discovered that they spontaneously found more situations in which to encourage not only the home-computing, but also their son's various other activities. During the first few days they tended to feel that after a working day, the two of them felt too tired to plan and execute supportive intervention strategies. Yet soon they found the task of expressing support easier, more spontaneous, and less artificial.*

Intervention programs that train parents to support their children and to be more responsive to their needs and achievements are less demanding then programs that train parents to act as their children's teachers and tutors. However, some parents express resentment toward these less demanding programs, feeling a strong urge to take a more active role in their children's lives, and to attempt to introduce changes in areas of importance and value to them. For parents who feel they wish to devote greater time and energy than that necessary for general supportive interventions, tutoring to their disabled children's in home-computing may provide a challenging answer.

## Parents as tutors

The goal of this approach centers on training parents in how to work with their children on the computer, and how to carry out a prescribed curriculum. Training parents to tutor their children (i.e., to take the role of teacher or therapist to their children) is based on the well-accepted concept that the family comprises the most powerful educational delivery system in the life of any child, in which parents may be viewed as the "primary teachers" of their children. Many parents of disabled children have been provided with special curricula and trained to tutor their disabled children in learning and communication areas. These trends reflect an important recognition of parental rights and abilities, and the increasing professional responsiveness to parents' wishes to be more actively involved in their children's education (Allen & Stefanowski-Hudd, 1987).

Computer time at school has been clearly shown to comprise a limited resource. Children have, legitimately, often expressed their feeling that if more computer time was available to them, a more skilled performance would be attainable. For handicapped children this situation has more serious implications, considering that children with disabilities require longer periods of learning and training in order to develop competent performance, and supportive parental practices usually do not suffice to meet the profound needs of these children for tutoring and assistance. Through the efficient integration of home-computing, parents can, in part, compensate for the acute lack of adequate computer time in the schools for their children with special needs. In order to apply home-computers effectively, parents can be trained to tutor their children in the use of academic software programs (e.g., teaching them written communication) with which the children have either not had previous contact, or to which they have already been exposed at school, but need additional time in order to master.

Training parents to tutor their children introduces changes not only to the role of parents, but also to various aspects of parent-child interactions. In order to develop an effective training model for the parental tutoring role, results from research on parental involvement in their children's schools, and on parent-child experiments and observations with and without computers, will be presented and discussed. In general, parent-child interactions can be regarded as the sharing of subjective understandings of the material and social environment. During tutoring, these interactions have an even more important influence on determining the level of the information provided, together with the social and parental experience to which a child is likely to be exposed, which may have a direct impact on the child's growth and development. The study of interactions and communication during tutoring is composed of two major interrelated factors: the partners' characteristics and the situational context (Fraser, 1986).

## Characteristics of the partners

The traditional unidirectional model of parent-child interactions posits that parents' behavior affects children's behavior and that fathers' and mothers' use of highly demanding teaching strategies (e.g., asking questions, providing explanations, etc.) predicts children's mental development (Hess, Holloway, Dickson, & Price, 1984). However, several studies have demonstrated that children's characteristics, such as gender (Block, 1983) and communicative status (Pellegrini, Brody, & Sigel, 1985), clearly influence parents' teaching styles.

Pellegrini, Brody, and Sigel (1986) examined factors affecting parents' teaching strategies, identifying and evaluating the effectiveness of different teaching strategies for engaging communicationally handicapped children in various tasks. Results indicated that parents varied their teaching strategies according to both task and children's communication status. Parents were also found to use different strategies with their handicapped and nonhandicapped children, using less demanding and more supportive strategies for the handicapped children.

It should be emphasized that although the parents used very different strategies for each group, the two groups of children were equally active participants in the tasks. More parental direction was necessary in order to actively involve the handicapped group. Thus, the communicationally handicapped group seemed less competent in the tasks, because they required more adult direction to sustain engagement. The results differentiated between "low demand" (e.g., statements, conversational management, turns) and "high demand" (e.g., questions) teaching strategies. The "low demand" strategies were shown to be rather effective in engaging the handicapped group, whereas the "high demand" strategies were effective only with the more competent children.

This orientation has been articulated by Vygotsky's (1978) notion of the zone of proximal development. The zone of proximal development was defined by Vygotsky as the difference between a child's actual level of independent problem solving and his/her potential level as determined by adult guidance of the child's behavior. According to this concept, parents' teaching style is governed by children's competence level and by the demands on children presented in a specific task.

The results of several studies which focus attention on parents with disabled children (Cunningham, Reuler, Blackwell & Deck, 1981; Eheart, 1982; Mahoney & Powel, 1988; Stoneman, Brody, & Abbott, 1983) confirm the zone of proximal development concept. They reported that these parents tended to match the information that they provided their children with the children's communicative and developmental level. As described earlier, in these families, parental style of interaction tended to be less responsive and more directive than that of parents of nondisabled children. This consistent finding has special importance, considering that, through adult-child teaching dialogues, adults instruct children in planning and guiding their own behavior. Such adult-directed teaching strategies play a necessary role in this model, if children are to become self-directed problem solvers. However, parental teaching strategies may often result in slowing the children's development toward becoming autonomously active and efficient problem solvers, and in further fostering their passivity and dependence. Studies of family climate among families with disabled children pinpointed interest at the unique interactional and communicational aspects, reporting that in these families, an increased emphasis on control was found, and less opportunities were available for the open expression of emotions (Margalit & Heiman, 1986).

A review of parent training outcomes (Dumas, 1984) further indicated that children's and even infants' characteristics were found to affect their parents' communications and interactions. Hanzlik and Stevenson (1986) found that mentally retarded infants were less responsive, and thus engaged in less behavior overall and in less verbal interactions. Their mothers were more active, using more commands than mothers of nondisabled infants, and the disabled infants were less active than the nondisabled peers. These results corroborated Hanzlik and Stevenson's (1986) concept of the lower limiting control strategy, which states that if infant behaviors are not emitted frequently enough according to maternal expectations, the mother attempts to elicit more frequent child behavior through prompts and directives. The mothers of disabled infants used more commands and more directive than responsive communication in an attempt to prompt more desired behaviors (Hanzlik & Stevenson, 1986).

## Situational contexts

The second factor postulated to play a major role in the study of interactions and communication during tutoring consists of the situational context (Fraser, 1986). Parents consistently use different teaching strategies in different contexts, reflecting more and less demanding tasks (Pellegrini, Brody, & Sigel, 1986; Sigel & McGillicuddy-DeLisi, 1983). The aforementioned research results demonstrated that parents' teaching styles were guided by children's level of competence in specific tasks.

In order to investigate the differences in the interactional styles related to different contexts and tasks, two types of activity were studied. A number of differences in parent-child interactional style have been demonstrated in the following two contexts: a book-reading activity and a home-computer activity involving an alphabet program (Worden, 1985; Worden, Kee, & Ingle, 1987). The level of verbal interaction was found to be lower in the computer activity. Book reading elicited overall more verbalization, and was more exclusively tutorial with respect to naming objects. Computer interactions featured more comments about objects, a greater number of parental directives about how to operate the computer, and more questions from the children.

These results require further studies detailing the specific characteristics of the computer context which are less encouraging of verbalized interaction, limiting it to directions and technical explanations. Parents' sensitization to this tendency focuses attention on attempting strategies that avoid a decrease in verbalization, such as: talking prior to and following computer performance, but refraining from talking during activity; reporting on details of the activity to a family member who was not present; asking the child to tutor another family member; or encouraging the child to verbalize effective strategies in ways that will help other family computer users.

## Objections and criticisms

The impact of the parent-as-teacher model on the parent-child relationship has also been debated and criticized. One can argue that the parent may gain satisfaction and confidence from teaching activities that promote the child's development, which in turn may favorably affect the parent-child relationship. However, professionals raised several objections to the training of parents for a teaching role, emphasizing the fact that parents can be frustrated and feel tense if the child shows little progress. Training parents to take over professional functions that are not usually present in their repertoire often makes them feel uncomfortable. A lifestyle and circumstances which afford the time and energy to consistently follow through on the child's teaching program are also essential.

Any parent who has attempted to assist his/her child with homework has probably encountered some of the risks and difficulties inherent in the role of parental tutor (e.g., parental anger at the child for the slow pace at which s/he grasps what the parent is trying to teach; children's feelings of frustration, anger, and of being insulted; parents' sense of helplessness when the lesson is unsuccessful or ends in tears). Horner (1987) listed several reasons for his objection to encouraging and advising parents of learning disabled children to tutor their own children. Horner's caution was related to the variability of the parents' teaching skills and to the guilt feelings expressed at times when parents found they were unable to provide help. Another aspect that should be considered consists of the parents' lack of free time. They already feel very tired and overburdened by their increased caring duties due to the child's disability. In addition, the parents' preoccupation with tutoring obligations may inhibit them from becoming involved in other ways in their children's lives. When parent-child interactions take on the character of teaching and "work," spontaneous and mutually enjoyable activities, or fulfillment of other parental functions, may be pushed aside.

Rodger (1986), highlighting issues derived from both the literature and clinical experience, criticized some of the assumptions made by professionals concerning parents' ability to be intensively involved with therapeutic programs for their handicapped children. Thus, he questioned whether professionals who trained parents to teach their disabled children are expecting too much of parents, who already may be physically and emotionally stressed by their childcare demands. Within the trend of giving parents more responsibilities, he discussed the possibility that the pendulum has swung too far and too rapidly in the new direction of allocating more responsibilities and duties to parents, causing these parents, whose time is consumed by the care of the disabled child, to feel guilty if they do not take on these additional obligations. Rodger suggested that professionals need to increase their awareness of the overall effects on parents of this additional responsibility. He questioned whether these professionals are being realistic in their demands and expectations from parents, who are first and foremost caregivers and parents and only then can attempt to be teachers and therapists.

Horner (1987) recommended that parents attempt not to teach academic curricula through tutoring, but rather to concentrate on areas that are more related to parental roles and functioning in the family environment, such as independent work habits and efficient problem solving techniques.

## Parents as tutors: An experiment

In order to demonstrate the intervention model, a description will be provided of one of the parent groups that were conducted in Tel-Aviv University (Margalit, Rochberg & Greenberg, 1988). This parent group was trained during six meetings to tutor their disabled children in a typing software.

### Sample

The participants in the pilot study consisted of 18 families (14 fathers and 10 mothers). In six families, the two parents participated together at each meeting, and one of the fathers even brought a nondisabled sibling (aged 11) as a support. All of the parents in the group owned computers at home, wanted to use the software being used at their children's school or social club, and were motivated to be more involved in their children's out-of-home-computing. Some of the parents possessed extensive professional knowledge in the area of computers, whereas others had merely purchased a computer without knowing how to use it or even what to do with it. No attempt was made to establish a homogeneous parental group, as this type of intervention constituted a completely new area of research requiring a qualitative case study method. The children, with mild disabilities such as learning disabilities and educable mental retardation, ranged in age from 8 to 14 years old.

### Method

The pilot intervention combined monthly group meetings and weekly telephone contacts for the duration of six months. The two group leaders were psychologists with vast experience in special education. Each leader maintained closer contact with nine families, including the weekly telephone contacts.

Each monthly meeting consisted of three sections:

1 A technical-informative session.
2 A theoretical presentation.
3 Counseling discussions.

In the first portion of each meeting, the technical-informative session, parents were trained in how to use a software program that had been developed at Tel-Aviv University to enhance keyboard typing and writing skills. Although this software was being taught and used at the time in the children's schools, these handicapped children often felt they lacked sufficient time to practice its usage.

In the second stage, the theoretical aspects of successful skill learning, information processing, and problem solving were presented, as related to the children's difficulties and to their performance with and without computers. It should be emphasized that the theoretical input was geared to increasing parents' understanding and to sensitizing them to the children's needs for tutoring and reinforcement in effective problem solving strategies, where the computer was used as a tool to help the children experience these processes. The children's school training followed this orientation, and it was deemed essential to teach parents the same vocabulary and self-instructional procedures that the children were tutored to use in school. Concepts from cognitive psychology and behavioral modification were discussed during this section, as related to the children's specific needs. The theoretical input was provided in order to increase parental involvement and support in the children's activities at their schools.

Counseling discussions, comprising the third section of the monthly meetings, pinpointed expressions and clarifications of parental difficulties and feelings (e.g., satisfaction, frustration) as related to the tutoring of their children. Parents raised questions and dilemmas that, although directly related to teaching their children, at the same time reflected their everyday difficulties with their children. Several parents detailed successful strategies for facilitating independent performance among their children, whereas others reported and complained about difficulties and frustrations.

Parents were trained to tutor their children using the software at least three times a week. The group leaders explained to the parents that this was an opportunity for parents to model an effective learning process for their children, by showing them how they learn, use a manual, follow directions in sequence, etc. Parents were asked to delay initiation of the training of their children until achieving a sense of familiarity and mastery of the software themselves. The training program applied Dik's (1984) conclusion that demonstrated the importance of parents' prior learning of basic computer skills until reaching a level of mastery, in order to empower the process of teaching their children.

## Observations and results

Parents shared their experiences and difficulties with other parents during the meetings and with the group leader in the telephone conversations. The following observations were reported by parents:

All of the children were very excited when the parents returned from the first meeting with the software. They were very eager to use the software at home. Parents' initial responses included:

> *"The children were very happy with the program. It was as if they were meeting with an old friend."*
>
> *"My daughter works better with the program than does any other family member, and she is very proud of that. So am I."*
>
> *"We got very good scores." Parents use of the plural "we" reflected their feelings of joint effort and pride.*

At first, some of the children worked with the software for hours; however, after a few days, several children developed an avoidance attitude similar to their behavior in other academic subjects. Their parents expressed extreme frustration that the children viewed the program as "just another" type of homework activity and treated it in a similarly rejecting manner, as they typically treated any homework assignment. Parents often debated regarding the most appropriate strategy: to force their children to learn the software, or to accept their refusal to be trained. Many times, the children preferred games, and the parents felt annoyed. Several mothers expressed their irritation that the children agreed to learn the software only in the presence of the parent. When these mothers tried to go to another room, their children stopped working. In one home it took the mother six weeks before her 11-year old dyslectic daughter agreed that she would continue to work independently even if her mother went into the kitchen.

In five families only the fathers were involved; in four families only the mothers were involved; and in the remaining families no clear division of responsibility with regard to home-computing was reported. The families regarded the child's activity with the computer as important, and some children used this attitude as a means to acquire more parental attention and support, by calling for more help and attention when working on the computer. The parents of these children expressed a concern that, through the computer usage, their children would increase their dependence on the parents.

As time progressed, parental involvement decreased, and parents began complaining about their role overload and their fatigue after a long working day. They described their impatience with their children's slow advancement and attempts to receive more attention. The pilot group's aim had not been defined as emotional sharing and/or providing an outlet for anger; however, dynamic interrelations between the group members began to develop. Several parents tended to criticize those parents who continued to report that they devoted time to teaching their children and that their efforts were successful, but the group fully supported those parents who expressed frustration, anger, and helplessness. As a result, the "successful" parents required continuous support and reinforcement from the group leaders, and emotional clarification of the negative expressions was necessary.

During the discussions, fathers and mothers alike tried to blame the quality of the software for their difficulties, and to provide their children with various additional academic software programs. They were helped in their search for new software programs by the group leaders. However, when the same demands for parental consistency in teaching became evident, and when the same difficulties in children's motivation were reported, several parents expressed their bitter disappointment from the lack of a miraculous impact from the training.

Several parents were very successful, continually reporting on their children's satisfaction from increased mastery. These parents also revealed pride in their children's improving ability to type homework on the computer and to prepare school projects -- a truly significant change for disabled children (e.g., one learning disabled boy with unreadable handwriting). One mother who reported that she began leaving secret letters to her daughter on the computer, conveyed her appreciation of another mode to communicate with her child.

Paradoxically, regardless of the frustrations reported by several parents, these same parents kept demanding a continuation of the meetings and telephone calls. Their attendance was prompt and consistent, and during the meetings they experimented with ways of supporting and reinforcing their children's computer-related activities. Eventually they began to feel that their initial expectations for their children's extensive training and for a miracle therapy were not realistic. Slowly, they began developing a more modest mode of parental involvement and support.

During the meetings, parents discussed shared topics related to home-computing, which also reflected common problems similar to those mentioned by parents in other parent groups, such as: (a) children's initially high level of motivation to invest great effort and patience in new areas (such as new software) but the difficulty of maintaining such motivation for long periods; (b) how to emphasize success for children who were often easily frustrated; and (c) how to encourage curiosity and explorative behavior in children who, in new situations, tend to be anxious, passive, and dependent in their behavioral style.

## Discussion

Parents' and children's individual differences were continuously emphasized. Some parents were able to devote much time to the home-computing and enjoyed teaching their children, whereas others were only able to support and reinforce desired activities. Some children learned very quickly and were able to present typed homework to their parents, while others developed rare talents for excuses and avoidance of various kinds of duties. Some children enjoyed computer games, while others loathed them. Most fathers found the computer an enjoyable activity to share with the disabled child, and some mothers reported similar attitudes.

A special subject that must be considered in every intervention program consists of the ambivalent manner with which parents often treated the subject of involvement and of tutoring their children. On the one hand, they wanted to be involved and active in their children's education. However, on the other hand, they resented playing such an overdemanding role and expressed feelings of fatigue, thus emphasizing an increased need for professional support (Hanline & Halvorsen, 1989). In the pilot parent group described above, several parents demonstrated their ambivalence by constantly reporting their difficulties and explaining why they were not able to work with their children on the software, yet demanding a continuation of the parent training.

## Conclusions

The conclusions of the literature reviewed and of the present qualitative pilot study pinpoint the need to develop different types of parental involvement, as a reply to individual differences among parents and children. A single model of parental tutoring may fit one family, but will be rejected as a complete mistake in other homes or in different ecological systems. The theoretical survey demonstrated the need for a two-strategy (i.e., support and tutoring) model for parental training, which will account for parental difficulties and will aim to:

1 Guide parents in their efforts to support and to teach their children.
2 Help adapt the most effective strategy to the partners' characteristics and to changing situational conditions.

The major issues for such guidance concern sensitizing parents to identify and be responsive and supportive to (a) children's needs in their home-computing and (b) available parental resources. Parents must learn to modify strategies in a flexible manner in order to adapt them to changing needs and conditions.

Further studies are necessary to explore methods of computer integration into homes of disabled children, with and without the external support of experts. It is of special interest to investigate whether parental involvement in home-computing will differ between families of children with and without special needs.

Ecological studies on the one hand, and experimentations among different kinds of parent groups on the other, may be used together to enrich our knowledge of effective, varied methods for counseling parents in assisting their handicapped children. The fulfillment of the new technologies' promises for these children and their families, and the development of parental roles in supporting these processes, call for extensive research in home-computing for special needs children. In order to support the prospect of a potential new role for fathers and mothers, attempts should be directed toward modeling and experimenting with different types of parent-child interactions.

In line with the theories of support, the goals of intervention programs for parents of disabled children can be viewed as aiming to (a) alter the parents' appraisals of current resources, (b) improve the parents' use of current resources, (c) improve the quality of supportive interactions within the family, (d) increase the resources available to the parent, and/or (e) reduce supportive resources' vulnerability to depletion or disruption (Vaux, & Athanassopulous, 1987). In order to achieve these goals, counseling strategies should not focus on the handicapped child and the disabling conditions in isolation, but rather must consider the total family unit, the complexity of the family dynamics, and the compensatory adjustments made by the parents and disabled child (Werth & Oseroff, 1987). A case study presentation of one family's attempts at effective computer integration via parental empowerment, may best illustrate the issues expounded throughout this section.

# 12

# Case Study: Danny R.

This chapter aims to present a case study to exemplify the integrative interventional model developed for parental involvement in the home-computing of their disabled children. The model evolved on the basis of the comprehensive literature reviewed in the field of computer technology integration into special education, and in light of parents' potential abilities and limitations as revealed by research on the stressors and resources available in families with disabled children. The case study of Danny R. will attempt to illustrate the different aspects of the suggested intervention model for empowering parents in their support and tutoring of their learning disabled children. The name of the child and demographic details of the family have been modified to protect their confidentiality, although the relevant facts remain faithful to the original data. The parents were trained by a special educator with vast experience working with children and families and presently specializing in computer applications for special education. Through attending to (a) the child's needs in terms of specific difficulties, and (b) the parents' expectations from technology, personal capacities, and difficulties, an attempt was made to identify the child-parent interactional patterns in Danny's family, to sensitize Danny's parents to processes and consequences, and to encourage a dynamic approach that would foster the child's growth and increased independence.

## Danny's diagnosis and referral

Danny, a 12-year-old male student, was diagnosed by the school psychologist, upon entering elementary school, as a learning disabled boy with average intelligence and sensori-motor difficulties. At age 12, Danny's difficulties were focused on the written communication area. The formal reason for the parents' request for consultation was his incredible number of spelling errors, not only when writing a free composition, but even when copying a short text. Danny's parents were extremely annoyed by his spelling difficulties and by the slow pace of his performance in academic and nonacademic tasks. They especially expressed their concern with his extremely slow pace of writing. Danny's handwriting was readable, but not very neat, suggesting a history of sensori-motor coordination difficulties. His teacher reported that Danny was often unable to finish writing out the instructions for his homework or to copy a few lines from the blackboard in the amount of time that proved sufficient for his classmates. However, he ignored the teacher's encouragement to work more quickly, or else was not able to follow up on that suggestion.

## The family system

Danny's father, an electrical engineer, aged 39, expressed his frustrations and disappointment from Danny's behavior at home. The second son, aged 9.4, was a successful student, especially talented in mathematics and natural studies, and shared with the father a mutual computer interest. Mr. R. often purchased and brought home new computer games and enjoyed playing with the younger son. A younger daughter, Miriam, aged 6, was the family's "little princess" whose beauty and cheerfulness everybody enjoyed.

The father even joked bitterly that Danny, being so slow and clumsy, was less successful at playing computer games than his little first-grade sister. Mr. R. wished to be able to have better interrelations with Danny, yet the father remarked that they presently had nothing in common, and that they rarely talked, except for Mr. R.'s sarcastic remarks about Danny's slow performance.

The mother, aged 36, a fourth-grade teacher at the local elementary school, became very irritated by Danny's written communication difficulties, including his slow writing, multiple spelling errors, and attempts to avoid lengthy written tasks. His compositions were often extremely short and were described by different teachers as "sets of telegrams and puzzles." Danny's many spelling errors were inconsistent, where the same word would sometimes be spelled in several mistaken forms on the same page, as if he were not sensitive to the word's schematic pattern. When asked to correct spelling errors, Danny often ended up adding new ones.

Mrs. R. viewed Danny's writing difficulties as an additional expression of her son's problems in concentration and organization. He began enthusiastically performing many tasks but showed difficulty finishing any of them. Danny's room was a mess, and he left his belongings wherever he was sitting; thus he often spent much time searching for items such as keys, a lost shoe, or a notebook. The mother commented that Danny had recently developed some motivation to overcome his slowness in writing and his spelling difficulties, but that he felt the school's remedial teaching was boring and ineffective. He complained that the spelling strategies that were suggested to him at school even decreased his writing speed.

### Intervention goals

In the context of Danny's special needs as described by his teacher and parents, the goals for Danny's training were defined as: to increase writing speed and decrease the number of spelling errors, using general strategies and domain-specific strategies. It was recommended that Danny be trained to learn efficient methods for performing tasks in general, such as improved methods for concentrating, understanding instructions, and memorizing data, as well as specific spelling strategies related to developing attention to word schemata and grammar rules. Accepting the child's long history of frustrations related to handwriting, a computer was suggested as the tutoring tool.

Danny's mother was reluctant, saying that she still seldom used the home-computer, whereas Danny's father volunteered excitedly, announcing that this was a task that he would like to work on, as he believed that through the computer his child could be helped. At school, Danny worked on the computer twice a week, using mostly drill-and-practice programs in mathematics, yet he was not very successful, and the teacher felt that the programs were not suitable to his slow pace.

From the family climate perspective, it seemed that an additional goal of the training would be to reinforce better interrelations between father and son, yet it was also necessary to identify a specific role for the mother in order to avoid any deterioration in her currently good interactions with her son.

## The home-computing environment

The R. family owned a home-computer for several years, and six months before they began the intervention, they purchased IBM PS-2 hardware. Mr. R. had originally initiated the computer's purchase, thinking that "Nowadays, it's important for every household to own a computer, just like everyone has a TV set." As the computer was intended for all of the family members, it was placed in the living room. Special furniture was purchased to provide a comfortable environment for the computer user. Mr. R. regularly used the computer either for work or leisure activities. He enjoyed purchasing new software programs, especially games, for the family, and he expected all of the family members to use the computer. Mrs. R. did not share her husband's attitudes and expectations for the computer. Her uses of the machine were limited to occasional word-processing for personal correspondence.

Prior to the tutoring period, the parents were instructed to observe the home-computing behavior of the family members for one week. The mother volunteered to carry out the observations, and she was particularly reinforced to perform that role, in view of her repeated verbalizations that emphasized her sense of being an inactive participant in computer activities, who almost avoided the machine entirely. Through her role as observer, she remained a participant throughout the intervention, and was more involved in the planning, as well as in later follow up stages.

After a week of observations, Mrs. R. reported that the family members treated the computer as they did the television, in the sense that whenever one person in the family began to use the machine, others usually joined in. This pattern of computer use naturally encouraged game playing but constituted a hindrance to work uses which required privacy and greater concentration. Mrs. R. reported that the major user of the computer was the younger son, who often initiated contacts with his father by calling him to discuss a difficulty or share an interest. The father occasionally used the computer for his own needs, such as to type a letter or to relax with a new game. Mostly, the home-computing activity was used as a bridge for the companionship interrelations between the father and his second son.

The young sister showed her interest by observing the father-son activity. From time to time, she was invited to use a simple graphic program or to type new words that she learned at school. She did not try to operate the computer independently, but sometimes joined others and then tried to be more active. The mother herself did not use the computer that week, similarly to prior weeks. She said that, as usual, she was too busy and too tired to use the computer, expressing no specific interest in learning.

Only through the observations did it become fully clear that Danny did not join in the home-computing activity. From time to time he watched his father and two siblings from a distance. Whenever he hesitantly tried to approach them, expressing some interest or a wish to use the computer, they ignored him without even realizing their rejection. Sometimes when Danny attempted to approach the group, the father sent him on various errands, such as buying a newspaper, saying that it was annoying to see Danny observing them, seeming so helpless.

## Training principles and description

The aims of the training were (a) to teach Danny touch-typing on the keyboard, and (b) to increase his speed of performance. Emphasis was placed on attentive perception of the word schemata, using a Hebrew typing software consisting of meaningful words. The following tutoring principles were used:

1 *Informed training.* Each meeting began by stating the aims of the training: attempting to reduce spelling errors and increasing the speed of typing, writing, and other learning activities.

2 *Frequent training.* Danny's work schedule was fixed: one-hour meetings every other day. During the first stages of training, the father sat with him, tutoring and encouraging quick and accurate performance.

3 *Assessment.* Prior to training, and at the end of each training week, the father assessed his son's spelling level through typed and hand-written dictations of two different brief texts (of 70 words each) at Danny's reading levels.

4 *Cognitive training.* The father encouraged Danny to memorize the words and not to type them letter by letter. Specific strategies whose effectiveness for improving spelling performance had been demonstrated by research (Margalit & Rot, 1989), such as visualization, awareness of the number and sequence of letters, and overpronunciation of all of the written letters, were combined with repeated encouragement to increase writing and typing speed.

5 *Metacognitive awareness.* Danny increased his means for improving performance through self-questioning as in "How can I do better?" and through private positive monologues as in "I know that I can do it very well."

Danny's home-computing intervention was planned for the duration of a four-month period, consisting of three one-hour sessions per week. At the beginning of the intervention, both parents were trained in the use of cognitive and metacognitive strategies for advancing speed and spelling performance. Mr. R. played the active role in the strategy training, whereas Mrs. R. took on a more supportive role. The parents met with the special educator monthly for follow-up and feedback. The training period may be divided into three main units of time.

### Stage 1

During the first month, Danny demanded his father's close presence. He did not agree to work unless the father sat next to him and gave him his full attention. Two interesting developments followed:

The father felt annoyed with the child's overdependence and need for such close attention. He kept commenting on his son's "babyish" behavior, yet surprisingly he accepted it and sat with the boy, thus confirming his son's expectations. It should be emphasized that at times it seemed that Danny took advantage of his father's strong motivation and belief in the value of the computer-supported intervention. The interactions between father and son were typically directive, with Mr. R. telling his son what to do, and less using open questions and suggestions. Although the father was sensitized to the developmental meaning of such interactions, he explained that his behavior was the most natural consequential adult behavior stemming from such a child's passive and dependent behavior. When the father tested his son's limits by sneaking in some newspaper reading, saying that Danny was just copying letters and words that he already knew, the son immediately stopped typing and sat inactively, looking very sad and waiting for the father to notice.

The other two siblings became intrigued by the change in the family climate, and constantly tested its meaning for them. They often entered the living room, attempting to distract their father and trying to understand why their brother was suddenly receiving so much special attention. The little sister announced that the typing program could also help her, demanding to use the program and to receive the father's attention. As this program had been presented from the beginning as Danny's program, he was the only one in the family who could allow others to use it. The idea behind this therapeutic strategy was to empower the boy who initially felt helpless with regard to various software programs at school and at home, and who was unable to develop skilled performance. As the typing program was easy to master, with various levels of speed, here was a good chance for Danny to succeed, yet competition with his siblings may have interfered with his motivated performance. It was decided that only when Danny felt ready would it be suggested that he should teach his sister, who could also benefit from the typing program, thus developing Danny's sense of power and control.

Danny's brother also noticed that Danny received a specific time every other day for working on the computer, and the brother also demanded clear definitions of computer time for various usages. He tried to place conditions on his computer time and on the father's presence as had Danny, but the "tired" father agreed only to identify access to computer time for his younger nondisabled son, while remaining very uncooperative with regard to suggestions to sit with him. Mr. R. reminded his younger son that the mother's earlier observations had demonstrated that the father already often sat with him voluntarily.

Danny overtly ignored his siblings' interest but appeared to enjoy the new situation. He maintained attention at his computing task while his father offered various explanations to the siblings regarding Danny's training. He continued to demand the father's presence, and Mr. R. complained yet tried various tutoring strategies and father-son interaction styles, using more questions and fewer directive communications such as statements and directions. The father was constantly supported by the mother, who observed the interactions, expressing understanding and appreciation of the efforts by both participants. Danny also sought out his mother's support, proudly sharing with her the improvements in spelling and speed.

## Stage 2

The entrance into the second stage of the training was noted by Danny's suggestion that he needed more computer time in order to advance his typing abilities more quickly. The "tired" father agreed to that demand for increased time, yet insisted that the greater computer time did not mean more of the father's time. Danny agreed, claiming that he now felt more sure of himself and inviting the father to join him only at the end of each training period to show off his achievements.

The father happily took advantage of the opportunity and agreed to the new arrangement. The mother at this time worried that Danny was really testing his father's interest in his work and was waiting to see if his father would now spend less and less time with him. She was almost ready to "fight" Danny's struggle for his father's time and attention, when she was surprised to see her husband taking his newspaper and cup of coffee and going to watch Danny working, even when Danny had not demanded the father's attention. It seemed that the father now enjoyed the new father-son interrelations, especially when they were not forced upon him and when they did not reflect Danny's increased dependency. It was interesting that Danny invested more and more time in the software program. He repeated spelling tests various times, recording only his best scores. He attempted to find periods when the father was not present, to continue experimenting, and thus to surprise him with new achievements.

## Stage 3

The third stage in the training was characterized by a more flexible and generalized attitude toward the different tasks which comprised the goals' for Danny's training:

1 Speed
2 Orderliness
3 Games
4 Maturity
5 Spelling

With regard to speed training, Danny now performed various academic and nonacademic tasks at a quicker rate. The specific reason for his earlier slowness remained unclear. Danny's slowness may have reflected anxiety and feelings of helplessness, but also the lack of skilled performance due to early sensori-motor difficulties. The mother also mentioned that she and her husband may have unintentionally tended to encourage slow performance by saying "do it slowly but surely." It is clear that through training Danny was able to develop a skilled and rapid typing performance and to appreciate the advantages of speed. He also increased the quantity and frequency of his writing and experimented more with words and sentences, achieving a more fluent writing performance. The teacher appreciated his new ability to finish writing on time, not to mention his quicker writing and typing. At home Danny was able to finish homework earlier, and enjoyed a sense of satisfaction from his more rapid performance.

Danny was constantly reinforced for the neatness and orderliness of his writing and typing. Soon he found it difficult to work in an environment with many distracting stimuli, and he expressed his sense of easiness with the computer, where only the task at hand appeared before his eyes. His parents were surprised when Danny arranged his room more neatly, telling his brother, who shared the room with him, that he could not concentrate with so many "things" on his desk.

Regarding computer games, Danny, to his father's and brother's delight, gradually became more and more interested in developing skilled performance in playing computer games. As the typing program which Danny used included several easy games that he was able to perform, he asked his father and his brother to introduce him to more difficult and challenging games. His quicker pace and positive experiences with the easy games included in the typing software enabled him to attempt faster "real" games. His father readily offered to teach him effective play strategies, and a shared interest and companionship was quickly developed between all the male members of the family, including Danny.

Danny's more mature behavior was demonstrated by his volunteering to teach his younger sister the typing software that he called "my program." He seemed to relate to the computer independently and more readily, reflecting a more mature approach to task performance.

Danny still showed a few spelling mistakes, but he had developed a sensitivity to errors that enabled him to stop writing and correct them. His teacher remarked on a significant improvement in Danny's written communication.

## Results

The results of the pre-post training assessments for spelling errors and speed are presented on Figure 12.1. Danny's increased accuracy and speed are evident in each of the three different texts that were presented before and after training. Even though different levels of difficulty were demonstrated for each of the three texts, the improved performance is demonstrated.

A discussion with the parents revealed that at the end of the tutoring period they were more satisfied not only with Danny, but also with themselves. The mother described Danny's achievements not only in terms of academic achievements, demonstrating a better ability for written communication, but also in more generalized terms, reflecting more mature behavior and closer relations with the father.

The father talked jokingly about periods of despair and overload, detailing how bored he had been with the necessity of sitting with Danny and devoting all his attention to encouraging his son's experimentations with the computer. However, he proudly reported that Danny's increased interest in computers had even evolved to the level of Danny's participating in afternoon computer courses, where he shared

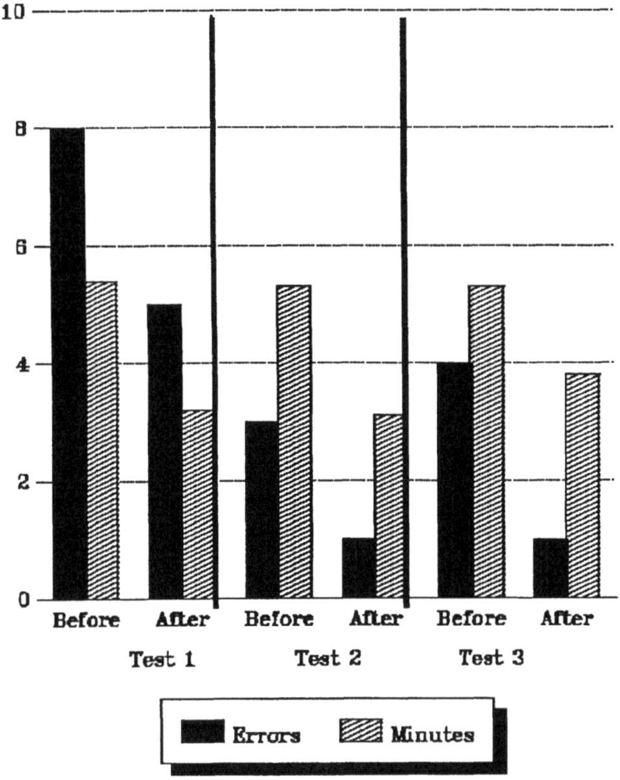


Figure 12.1. Danny R.'s pre- and post-training scores for spelling errors and speed

that interest not only with his father and brother, but also with peers.

The father summarized the impact of the training as not only helping his child (who recently insisted to teachers that he will now present typed homework and projects instead of writing them), but also empowering the father in his support of the child's home-computing which had been used to overcome an academic difficulty.

It should be remembered that Danny is a learning disabled child. His father used the computer to help him in a specific area of academic and behavioral difficulty, and thus developed a unique father-son interaction. The parents acknowledged the fact that new school demands and age-related tasks may result in new difficulties for Danny in the future. However, they felt more ready for new challenges and more able to help their children. Mrs. R. revealed that before training, although she felt that Mr. R. was a very supportive husband, she was constantly worried due to the increased responsibility of caring for Danny's special needs. Now the two parents expressed the sense that they felt like an empowered and unified team, ready to help their children. Although no direct intervention was applied in Danny's family regarding areas of future concern for his adjustment, the changes evidenced in this family clearly empowered them to better confront future difficulties.

## Conclusions

The current case study exemplified the integration of the computer in a home where it was already in use. The disabled child may find difficulty in participating in the family's home-computing, and special support and tutoring may be necessary to assist the child in becoming more adaptatively involved in computer activity. Parents' training, when they want and are able to tutor their children, focuses on the training procedures emphasizing metacognitive awareness and the parent-child interactional style.

Home-computing intervention programs have been developed along these two patterns of support and tutoring, assuming that individual adaptation is essential in order to match the programs and training to parents' and children's characteristics and to familial circumstances (Dumas, 1984). In line with Helm and Kozloff's (1986) demonstration of the shortcomings in several parent training programs for families of handicapped children, where these groups were reported as typically helping families only with respect to a limited number of their short-term needs, the present model attempted to address individualistic and systemic aspects in the planning. Research related to major aspects of parent-child interactions, such as the participants' characteristics and the contexts' characteristics, were considered for families with disabled children.

The aforementioned case study exemplified the fact that intervention programs which train parents to support their children, and to be more responsive to their needs and achievements, may affect interactions between all of the family members, improving attitudes and behavioral tendencies toward the disabled child. Subtle modifications in parent-child and nondisabled-disabled sibling interactions which result from such supportive computer integration strategies have the potential for significantly influencing the family relationships, thus increasing the quality of life for the disabled child and his/her entire family system. The parents' (and sometimes siblings') joint participation in such a positive experience as bolstering and witnessing the disabled child's increased self-confidence and ability not only in academic competence areas but also in computer technology, a field considered at the forefront of modern development, can change attitudes and lessen the stress experienced by families with disabled children.

# Section IV

## Epilogue: Disabilities, Technology, and Families

# 13

# Summary and Future Directions

The overall intent of this volume was to provide a model for empowering parents in their support of their children's home-computing. As such, the text focused on providing a relatively compendious overview of the literature dealing with three main subjects areas:

1 Effective integration of technology for children with mild disabilities.
2 Stress, resources, coping, and needs for support among the families of these children.
3 Parent-child interactions and major strategies for supportive programs.

The first section of the text provided a foundation for the present model, through a comprehensive review of research, pinpointing attention at the various topics in which the schools' integration of technology played an important role in fostering the development and achievements of children with mild disabilities. In the current model, children may achieve a level of automaticity in their performance of basic skills through drill-and-practice software training programs. The children's writing skills can be advanced through specific instruction in wordprocessing, while their effective problem solving skills may be developed using metacognitive training integrated with computer games and simulations.

It should be emphasized that the research surveyed in the first section clearly highlighted the crucial role played by significant adults and by appropriate instructional procedures in the effective usages of computers as a tool to facilitate the educational process. The naive belief that the simple introduction of technology will affect the life of these children has been rejected, while the central role of teachers and of curriculum-based procedures, as would be implemented in non-computerized instruction, was accentuated in the planning of technology-supported instruction.

In addition, the need for disabled and nondisabled children's increased computer time and access was addressed by several studies that criticized the schools' attempts at the integration of technology, especially in relation to the children's insufficient time and exposure to the impact of the technology. In contrast, home-computing appears to provide greater computer time. Despite the acknowledgement of the fundamental role played by adults, such as teachers, in the adaptation of technology to children's educational performance, research on the home-computing of disabled children remains in its early stages, and the role of parents in supporting their children's home-computing has yet to be comprehensively investigated.

Before attempting to identify effective parental strategies for supporting the home-computing of their children, a survey of the research on families with disabled children was presented in Section 2. The survey attempted to clarify these parents' abilities and difficulties in accepting a new computer-supportive role, as an addition to their already existing pressures. Different sources of family stress were described as interrelated and as affecting the family's growth and functioning: The emotional stress stemming from the pain and distress of having a disabled child and the stress resulting from the increased childcaring burden due to greater demands on the family resources. The father's role was reported as having a unique contribution to children's development; however, among families with disabled children fathers often tended to accept the role of mother's helper, thus neglecting to define a unique paternal role.

In order to empower parents, effective coping strategies were identified and studied, and the role of meaningful support networks was highlighted. Parents' struggle in their development of new roles, and in their abilities to reorganize family resources to meet increased needs, were surveyed. A discussion of family climate and patterns of parent-child interactions were identified through various research methods, and the fathers' and mothers' tendency to develop a directive, dominating interactional style, as an effective solution to the children's distractible, passive, and helpless behavior patterns, was reviewed.

Research reported that such parent-child interactional patterns failed to facilitate development and adjustment in disabled and nondisabled children alike. From these results emerged the realization of the need to sensitize parents to interactional aspects of their support for their children. Alternative modes of interaction, with parents using questions and discussions instead of statements and commands, were found to exist in the repertoire of these parents. However, counseling and training appear essential in order to help parents include such interaction patterns spontaneously. Additional studies should be conducted to clarify interrelations between critical aspects of deficient information processing of children with mild disabilities (Reschly, 1987), and to identify the role of parent-child interactions in fostering or delaying the children's development and thus in affecting various aspects of remedial work.

The results of several surveys were delineated in order to illustrate the process of the computer's entrance into these homes. Parental expectations for a magic impact on needs in critical areas were contrasted with the different styles developed by families in their home-computing environments. Both mothers and fathers expected a significant change following the computer's introduction into the home, with the fathers placing special emphasis on the emotional meaning of the computer, thereby centering responsibility for their children's improvement on the machine itself. However, moving from expectations to practices, in only a few homes were fathers or mothers able to take an active role in supporting their children and in using the computing as a bridge between the school- and home-computing environments. Most parents felt that they had fulfilled their contributions and roles by simply providing their children with the computer.

## The parent empowerment model

The supportive computer-integration model presented in the text reflected an *individualistic, dynamic* approach to the *empowering* of parents in assisting their children:

*Empowering* constituted the foundation of the model developed, in light of the parents' simultaneous desire for involvement and difficulty in actually becoming involved. On the one hand, parents revealed a wish to feel coherent and effective, and to be active in affecting the lives of their disabled as well as nondisabled children. On the other hand, the stress resulting from parents' pain, sorrow, and overload of duties impaired their effectiveness and self-assurance. The integration of technology into the home seems to develop a context for fulfilling the three basic aspects of empowering parents (Dunst & Trivette, 1987). Home-computing may be considered an area for these parents to demonstrate their capacity to become competent (and some of them are already competent in computer technology), to have enabling experiences related to their disabled child, and thus to acquire a greater personal sense of control.

For many parents, and especially for fathers, using technology represented a promise of unique and challenging opportunities. When the technology, which appealed to them, was involved, parents felt they possessed abundant personal energy and a greater readiness to invest renewed efforts in helping their children.

*Individualistic* depicts the model, in the sense that the model presented accounted for the impact of individual differences during intervention planning. The realization, that the amount of personal investment that fathers and mothers can afford differed from family to family and from parent to parent, was highlighted as extremely important for any intervention planning. Realistic expectations from parents were deemed critical, including the acceptance of individual personality differences (e.g., in parental abilities to invest effort and time), the clarification of the subjective meaning of technology for each parent, and the investigation of these parents' overall life demands as proportionally related to family resources. It was emphasized that intervention plans which fail to consider the additional difficulties and demands constantly faced by these parents will be limited in their impact.

*Dynamic* described the model in several ways. In one sense, the model accounted for dynamic, periodic changes in the family lifecycle. As a rule it is extremely difficult for people to accept new, additional obligations that are time demanding for the duration of long periods. However, for specific periods, people are willing to introduce changes into their lifestyle and to devote seemingly unlimited time and energies toward a valuable cause. Understanding these periodic changes in the lives of individuals and families was considered crucial for effective intervention planning. The current model was also dynamic in the sense that a static objective for effective computer intervention did not serve as the focus of this model, but rather the procedural processes during the different stages of the intervention received great emphasis. The process-oriented dyamics involved in the home learning environment will be further explored below. Family dynamics, as in the role of constantly changing interrelationships between the various family members (e.g., parent-child and disabled-nondisabled sibling interactions), also constituted a central foundation of the conceptualization.

The two types of parental intervention suggested, direct tutoring and planned support, do not represent discrete groups of activities but rather rest on a continuum of parent-child interactions. Training parents to tutor their children can be viewed as an example of the most active and effective, but also the most tiring and time-consuming intervention. Those parents who wish to be trained as teachers of their children in a specific area, must realize the serious implications for their leisure time and everyday life. The parents studied often felt a sense of power and satisfaction from such an intensive investment as the computer-supported intervention, yet many of them found it difficult to continue such tutoring of their children over long periods of time. In addition, accepting the role of teachers for their children may negatively affect their ability to fulfill their roles as parents.

Planned support of the children's computing activities and the development of a learning environment at home were considered valuable in fostering the desired results and less personally demanding, but also less demonstrative in impact. Any attempt to empower parents, and not to distress them, requires careful planning in order to adapt demands to changing parental capacities, resources, and personal goals.

## Future directions

The home-computing of children with mild disabilities comprises a new field of research and clinical practice. Two major directions should constitute the focus of future research on home-computing: the interactions between school and home systems (i.e., between teacher and parent), and the interactions within the family environment. Environments affect family life, both influencing the capacity of parents to care for their children and having a direct impact on the children's adjustment. The ecology of human development involves the scientific study of the progressive mutual adaptation between a growing human being with as without disabilities, and the changing properties of the immediate settings in which the developing child lives (Bronfenbrenner, 1979). The distinguishing characteristics of the ecological perspective consists of its insistence on the holistic understanding of individuals and the environmental forces that affect them (Wharf, 1988). Issues such as characteristics of the home, optimal learning environments, and parent-teacher interrelation patterns must be studied in detail within the present ecological home-school interrelation perspective aimed at empowering the families.

## Teacher-parent interrelations

Central to the ecological orientation lies the concept of interrelationships between systems and between individuals within those systems (Pence, 1988). It is unanimously accepted that teachers need intensive training prior to introducing technology to their students in the school environment, and during its usage in the various types of remedial work. In order to extend the desired impact of technology to the home-environment, teacher training programs must address topics related to home-computing and to parent-teacher interrelations concerning the children's academic experience.

The importance of parents' involvement in their children's education has already been elaborated by various studies, yet a difficulty has often been revealed in developing meaningful, continuous interrelations between home and school. In many cases, fathers have generally tended to absent themselves from school programs that attempted to stimulate parental involvement in their children's school activities. Technology introduction provides a special context for meaningful interrelations, and as such, a challenge and an opportunity to appeal to parents and to train teachers, thereby building a bridge of new interrelations between school and home environments.

A key to the development of intervention programs consists of responsiveness to the needs and characteristics of the participants. It is assumed that the programs will develop a structure and a content which attracts and sustains the participants' involvement (Powell, 1988). Teacher-training programs that are presently being developed at Tel-Aviv University attempt to help teachers to empower parents in their abilities to promote their children's adjustment, integrating the following three main aspects:

1. Training teachers in effective computer integration for remedial teaching.
2. Sensitizing teachers to important aspects of family dynamics, parental stress, and the need for parental empowering in order to develop a meaningful bridge toward a continuum between school and home environments.
3. Training teachers to develop a partnership with parents, through effective introduction and usage of technology in the two environments.

Ecological studies are needed to investigate the impact of these programs, in which various direct and indirect influences may account for changes. Teachers may work directly with their students, but also may expand the impact of their work through parental training. Through the effective integration of technology in the children's curricula, parents and teachers can develop an interrelational partnership for fostering the children's development in academic and leisure activities. Comprehensive research into the meaning of the parent-teacher partnership for each participant, investigating expectations and goals of each partner, may direct the preparation of effective programs.

Another important question that deserves serious investigation concerns whether such a partnership of mutual interrelations can be developed only in the area of technology, as a direct answer to a new need, or whether these interactions may be generalized into various additional areas of children's learning. The novelty of the technology arena may serve to facilitate meaningful interrelations between teachers and parents with regard to computers, yet it remains to be seen as to whether such a partnership will remain limited and short-term, maintained only until the novelty of the new field disappears, or whether these relations may be fostered to evolve into a long-term, satisfying connection that will demonstrate important ramifications for the entire special educational process.

## Learning environments at home

Another important area that requires focused research efforts concerns the investigation of computer-assisted learning environments in homes. The home as the learning context must be carefully considered, in view of its own specific characteristics, which may facilitate or inhibit learning processes. Contexts control human behavior, and the individual's mindset determines the way in which particular contexts are interpreted (Langer, 1989). Within a goal-oriented context, typified by most intervention programs, the emphasis is placed on outcome (i.e., the disabled child's overcoming his/her areas of deficiency), thereby enabling the development of a mindless behavior pattern (e.g., the parents may adopt a directive, dominating communicational style, as described previously). For example, if people think they know how to handle a situation, they will not feel a need to pay attention to details. Just as mindlessness consists of the rigid reliance on old, familiar categories, mindfulness implies the continual re-creation of new ones.

A preoccupation with outcome can lead to mindlessness, whereas a process orientation intervention may be defined as mindfulness. A mindful state implies openness to new information and the active, continuous re-processing of elements within the learning environment. Process-oriented intervention programs may sensitize parents to various aspects of their behavior style which are related to fostering effective learning environments. In line with Cornell and Grossberg's conclusions, the most important aspects within the family context consisted not with what the parents do with the child, but rather how they do it. The optimal learning environment may be enhanced when learning processes are emphasized and when parents and children, together, learn new tasks, enjoy the challenge of overcoming difficult problems, and use effective problem solving strategies.

Such a learning environment implements a mindful approach to formulating effective procedures of learning processes, rather than accentuating specific contents and outcomes. In order for parents to allow for the effective integration of computer technology, the procedures used for technology-based training should receive as much consideration, if not more, than the specific objectives established for improving the disabled child's performance. Parents should be ever mindful of the dynamic procedural processes during training, rather than of the particular goal of the intervention.

The contextual impact was clearly demonstrated through the amount of change evidenced in the families of disabled children studied. In various families, the entrance of computers seemed to affect the interactional style of the family members, whereas in other homes, the existing family dynamics were further emphasized through the new addition to the family environment. Some families revealed significant modifications as a result of the impact of the technology integration, whereas others demonstrated almost no change. These findings substantiate the thesis stated in this text, that the computer introduction and usage cannot be expected to create significant results, unless the contextual features in which the technology is integrated are dynamic and open to change. In families which rigidly adhere to previous modes of behavior and interrelations, the computer's entrance into the home will only exacerbate or highlight the existing family context, such as role and power distribution.

In several homes, the computer was often used not only by the disabled child, but by all the family members. Within these family environments, a constant struggle for additional computer time was evident, and the structuring of family rules was necessary to enable appropriate and satisfying computer access to the different users within the family. In these homes, the children's extensive, wide range of home-computer usages was revealed. In other homes, a learning environment was enhanced through the introduction of new and stimulating software by parents or siblings. The siblings' new awareness and acceptance of the disabled child as a full-fledged participant in the family's home-computing activity carries strong weight in modifying the sibling relationships.

The support of older as well as younger siblings can be included in the potential resources available to families introducing the computer into their home. The acknowledgement of stages in the development of computer literacy (i.e., beginner's anxiety and needs for support and help), the sharing of excitement, feelings of mastery and interest, and the modeling of efficient problem solving through software learning, jointly contribute to the development of the effective learning environment at home.

The results of various observations and short-term experimentations have pinpointed the ability to change interrelations within the family context through a comprehensive, process-oriented, supportive intervention model of effective learning procedures based on parental guidance. The importance of parents' roles and of their ability to change their functions, especially concerning the unique paternal role which received emphasis throughout this text, deserve increased attention in future research. Research has yet to identify the critical factors within the family context that may contribute to facilitating the desired process of parental empowerment and children's development.

Differential parental roles should also constitute an area of research, with specific emphasis on the transactional aspects of the two parents' interrelations. If the father's potential role is expanded, how will the mother's functioning be affected? Will her relations with her child be impaired? How can both parents' roles be enhanced simultaneously and complementarily? The emphasis placed on the unique paternal role in this text can easily be generalized to any other family member, and most easily to the mother. Whoever in the family takes more instrumental functions upon himself or herself is likely to be the individual who will best be able to take advantage of the computer technology, empowering the parent to integrate the technology for the disabled child.

This volume has attempted to provide a model for empowering parents through their support of their disabled children's home-computing. As the literature presented in this volume attests, the intervention model has only reached its beginning stage, requiring clarification and intensive study to investigate the various aspects of technology's promises and families' stress and resources. The intensive study of the various interrelations aspects within the family system, and between systems is central to foster opportunities for parental empowerment. The use of technology as a bridge between the two important systems in the life of children --school and home -- constitutes a very promising and challenging topic for teachers and parents in their development of partnership patterns. Research should be directed toward developing detailed individualistic and dynamic modes of empowering interventions.

# References


Ackerman, P. L. (1987). Individual differences in skill learning: An integration of psychometric and information processing perspectives. *Psychological Bulletin, 102*, 3-27.

Alexander, P. A., & Judy, J. E. (1988, April). *The integration of domain-specific and strategic knowledge in academic performance.* Paper presented at the AERA Annual Convention, New Orleans, LA.

Allen, D. A., & Stefanowski-Hudd, S. (1987). Are we professionalizing parents? Weighing the benefits and pitfalls. *Mental Retardation, 25*, 133-139.

Anderson, J. R. (1983). *The architecture of cognition.* Cambridge, MA: Harvard University Press.

Anderson, J. R. (1985). *Cognitive psychology and its implications* (2nd ed). New York: Freeman.

Antonovsky, A. (1979). *Health, stress, and coping.* San Francisco: Jossey-Bass.

Antonovsky, A. (1987). *Unraveling the mystery of health.* San Francisco: Jossey-Bass.

Antonovsky, A., & Sourani, T. (1988). Family sense of coherence and family adaptation. *Journal of Marriage and the Family, 50*, 79-92.

Avison, W. R., & Turner, R. J. (1988). Stressful life events and depressive symptoms: Disaggregating the effects of acute stressors and chronic strains. *Journal of Health and Social Behavior, 29*, 253-264.

Bandura, A. (1977). Self-efficacy: Toward a unifying theory of behavior change. *Psychological Review, 84*, 191-215.

Bandura, A. (1978). The self system in reciprocal determinism. *American Psychologist, 4*, 344-358.

Bandura, A. (1982). Self-efficacy mechanism in human agency. *American Psychologist, 37*, 122-147.

Bandura, A., & Schunk, D. (1981). Cultivating competence, self-efficacy and intrinstic interest through proximal self-motivation. *Journal of Personality and Social Psychology, 41*, 586-598.

Bauer, J. A. (April, 1988). *An exploration of gender-related patterns of microcomputer use within 51 families.* Paper presented at the AERA Annual Convention, New Orleans, LA.

Becker, H. (1986). *Instructional use of school computers* (Issue 1). Baltimore: The Johns Hopkins University Center for Social Organizations of Schools.

Beishuizen, J. (1988). Microcomputers and skill development. In J. Beishuizen, J. Tobin, & P. R. Weston (Eds.), *The use of the microcomputer in teaching and learning*. Amsterdam: Swets and Zeitlinger.

Beit-Hallahmi, B. H. (1981). The kibbutz family revival or survival. *Journal of Family Issues, 2*, 259-274.

Bettelheim, B. (1969). *The children of the dream*. New York: Macmillan.

Block, J. (1983). Differential premises arising from differential socialization of the sexes: Some conjectures. *Child Development, 54*, 1354-1365.

Bos, C. S. (1988). Process-oriented writing: Instructional implications for mildly handicapped students. *Exceptional Children, 54*, 521-527.

Brandstatter, H. (1983). Emotional responses to other persons in everyday life situations. *Journal of Personality and Social Psychology, 45*, 871-883.

Bronfenbrenner, U. (1979). *The ecology of human development: Experiments by nature and design*. Cambridge, MA: Harvard University Press.

Bronfenbrenner, U. (1986). Ecology of the family as a context for human development: Research perspectives. *Developmental Psychology, 22*, 723-742.

Brown, A. L., Campione, J. C., & Day, J. D. (1981). Learning to learn: On training students to learn from texts. *Educational Researcher, 10*, 14-21.

Brown, A. L., & Campione, J. C. (1986). Psychological theory and the study of learning disabilities. *American Psychologist, 14*, 1059-1068.

Bruner, J. (1985, June/July). Models of the learner. *Educational Researcher, 14*, 5-8.

Burden, R., & Thomas, D. (1986). Further perspectives on parental reaction to handicap. *The Exceptional Child, 33*, 140-145.

Carey, R., & Gall, M. (1986). Patterns of microcomputer use at home and at school by secondary school students. *Educational Technology, 26*, 29-31.

Case, L. P., & Harris, K. R. (1988, April). *Self-instructional strategy training: Improving the mathematical problem solving skills of learning disabled students.* Paper presented at the AERA Annual Convention, New Orleans, LA.

Charles, R. I., & Lester, K., Jr. (1984). An evaluation of a process-oriented instructional program in mathematical problem solving in grades 5 and 7. *Journal for Research in Mathematical Education, 15*, 15-34.

Chiang, B. (1986). Initial learning and transfer effects of microcomputer drills on LD students' multiplication skills. *Learning Disabilities Quarterly, 9*, 118-123.

Christiansen, C., & Gerber, M. M. (1986). *Effects of game format in computerized drill and practice on development of automaticity in single digit addition for learning disabled students* (Tech. Rep. No. 20). Santa Barbara: University of California, Project TEECH.

Cirillo, S., & Sorrentino, A. M. (1986). Handicap and rehabilitation: Two types of information upsetting family organization. *Family Process, 25*, 283-292.

Clark, L. A., & Watson, D. (1988). Mood and mundane: Relations between daily life events and self-reported mood. *Journal of Personality and Social Psychology, 54*, 296-308.

Clarke-Stewart, K. A. (1978). And Daddy makes three: The father's impact on mother and young child. *Child Development, 49*, 466-478.

Cobb, S. (1976). Social support as a moderator of life stress. *Psychosomatic Medicine, 38*, 300-313.

Coe, D. E. (1988, April). *Emergent writing behavior of young children: Taking the task of writing to task.* Paper presented at the AERA Annual Convention, New Orleans, LA.

Cohen, S., & Waren, R. (1985). *Respite care: Principles, programs, and policies.* Austin, TX: Pro-Ed.

Cohen, S., & Wills, T. A. (1985). Stress, social support, and the buffering hypothesis. *Psychological Bulletin, 98*, 310-357.

Cole, D. A. (1986). Out-of-home placement and family adaptation: A theoretical framework. *American Journal of Mental Deficiency, 91*, 226-236.

Cornell, D. G., & Grossberg, I. W. (1987). Family environment and personality adjustment in gifted children. *Gifted Child Quarterly, 31*, 59-64.

Cosden, M. A., Gerber, M. M., Semmel, D. S., Goldman, S. R., & Semmel, M. I. (1987). Microcomputer use within micro-education environments. *Exceptional Children, 53*, 399-409.

Craig, K. (1987). Thinking and writing. *The Macintosh Lab Monitor, 3*, 12-14.

Crnic, K. A., Friedrich, W. N., & Greenberg, M. T. (1983). Adaptation of families with mentally retarded children: A model of stress, coping, and family ecology. *American Journal of Mental Deficiency, 88*, 125-138.

Crnic, K. A., Greenberg, M. T., Ragozin, A. S., Robinson, N. M., & Basham, R. B. (1983). Effects of stress and social support on mothers of premature and full-term infants. *Child Development, 54*, 209-217.

Cronkite, R. C., & Moos, R. H. (1984). The role of predisposing and moderating factors in the stress-illness relationship. *Journal of Health and Social Behavior, 25*, 372-393.

Cunningham, C. E., Reuler, E., Blackwell, J., & Deck, J. (1981). Behavioral and linguistic developments in the interactions of normal and retarded children with their mothers. *Child Development, 52*, 62-70.

Dalton, B. M., Morocco, C. C., & Neale, A. E. (1988, April). *"I have lost my story!": Mastering the machine skills for word processing*. Paper presented at the AERA Annual Convention, New Orleans, LA.

Dede, C., & Gottlieb, D. (April, 1984). *The long-term influence of home microcomputers on family/school relationships*. Paper presented at the AERA Annual Convention, New Orleans, LA.

Demos, E. S. (1988). Technological resources for parents. *Reading Horizons, 28*, 85-91.

Deno, S., Marston, D., & Mirkin, P. (1982). Valid measurement procedures for continuous evaluation of written expression. *Exceptional Children, 48*, 368-371.

Dik, D. W. (November, 1984). *Empowering parents through computer literacy training*. Paper presented at the National Adult Education Conference, Louisville, KY.

Dumas, J. E. (1984). Indiscriminate mothering: Empirical findings and theoretical speculations. *Advanced Behavior Research Therapy, 6*, 13-27.

Dunst, C. J., & Trivette, C. M. (1987). Enabling and empowering families: Conceptual and intervention issues. *School Psychology Review, 16*, 443-456.

Dyson, L., & Fewell, R. R. (1986). Stress and adaptation in parents of young handicapped and nonhandicapped children: A comparative study. *Journal of the Division for Early Childhood, 10*, 25-34.

Edyburn, D. L., & Lartz, M. N. (1987). The teacher's role in the use of computers in early childhood education. *Journal of the Division of Early Childhood, 10*, 225-263.

Eheart, B. K. (1982). Mother-child interactions with nonretarded and mentally retarded preschoolers. *American Journal of Mental Deficiency, 87*, 20-25.

Elliott-Faust, D. J., & Pressley, M. (1986). How to teach comparison processing to increase children's short- and long-term listening comperison monitoring. *Journal of Educational Psychology, 78*, 27-33.

Ellis, E., & Sabornie, E. (1986). Effective instruction with microcomputers: Promises, practices and preliminary findings. *Focus on Exceptional Children, 19*, 1-16.

Epstein, J. L. (1985). Home and school connections in schools of the future: Implications of research on parent involvement. *Peabody Journal of Education, 62*, 18-41.

Fais, L. (1987). Post-testing results and year-end observations. *The Macintosh Lab Monitor, 3*, 3-9.

Fernberg, P. M. (1985). Designing the workplace for the knowledge worker. *Modern Office Technology, 30*, 73-82.

Fitzgerald, G., Fick, L., & Milich, R. (1986). Effective instruction with microcomputers: Promises, practices and preliminary findings. *Focus on Exceptional Children, 19*, 376-379.

Flavell, J. H. (1981). Cognitive thinking. In W. P. Dickson (Ed.), *Children's oral communication skills* (pp. 35-60). New York: Academic Press.

Flavell, J. H. (1987). Speculations about the nature and development of metacognition. In F. E. Weinert, & R. H. Kluwe (Eds.), *Metacognition, motivation, and understanding* (pp. 21-29). Hillsdale, NJ: Lawrence Erlbaum.

Folkman, S., & Lazarus, R. S. (1980). An analysis of coping in a middle-aged community sample. *Journal of Health and Social Behavior, 21*, 219-239.

Folkman, S., & Lazarus, R. S. (1985). If it changes, it must be a process: Study of emotions and coping during three stages of college examination. *Journal of Personality and Social Psychology, 48*, 150-170.

Folkman, S., & Lazarus, R. S. (1988). Coping as a mediator of emotion. *Journal of Personality and Social Psychology, 54*, 466-475.

Folkman, S., Lazarus, R. S., Dunkel-Schetter, C., Delongis, A., & Gruen, R. J. (1986). Dynamics of a stressful encounter: Cognitive appraisal, coping, and encounter outcomes. *Journal of Personality and Social Psychology, 50*, 992-1003.

Folkman, S., Schaefer, C., & Lazarus, R. S. (1979). Cognitive processes as mediators of stress and coping. In V. Hamilton, & H. Warburton (Eds.), *Human stress and cognition processes* (pp. 265-298). New York: Wiley.

Fondacaro, M. R., & Moos, R. H. (1987). Social support and coping: A longitudinal analysis. *American Journal of Community Psychology, 15*, 653-673.

Fraser, B. C. (1986). Child impairment and parent/infant communication. *Child: Care, health and development, 12*, 141-150.

Frederick, C. M., & Wellborn, J. G. (1988, April). *Father involvement and its relationship to perceived competence and autonomy in elementary-age children.* Paper presented at the AERA Annual Convention, New Orleans, LA.

Frey, K. S., Fewell, R. R., & Vadasy, P. F. (1989). Parental adjustment and changes in child outcome among families of young handicapped children. *Topics in Early Childhood Special Education, 8*, 38-57.

Friedrich, W. N., Wilturner, L. T., & Cohen, D. S. (1985). Coping resources and parenting mentally retarded children. *American Journal of Mental Deficiency, 90*, 130-139.

Gallagher, J. J., Beckman, P., & Cross, A. H. (1983). Families of handicapped children: Sources of stress and amelioration. *Exceptional Children, 50*, 10-19.

Gerson, M. (1978). *Family, women, and socialization in the kibbutz.* Lexington, MA: Heath.

Giacquinta, J. B., & Lane, P. A. (April, 1988). *Obstacles to children's home academic microcomputing: An empirical test of a causal model.* Paper presented at the AERA Annual Convention, New Orleans, LA.

Gil, K. M., Keefe, F. J., Sampson, H. A., McCaskill, C. C., Rodin, J., & Crisson, J. E. (1987). The relation of stress and family environment to atopic dermatitis symptoms in children. *Journal of Psychosomatic Research, 31*, 673-684.

Glaser, R. (1984). Education and thinking: The role of knowledge. *American Psychologist, 39*, 93-104.

Goin, L. I. (1988, December). *Developing mathematical fluency in learning disabled students: From theory to practice.* Paper presented at the Annual CEC/TAM Conference on Special Education and Technology, Reno, NV.

Goldberg, S., Marcovitch, S., MacGregor, D., & Lojkasek, M. (1986). Family response to developmentally delayed preschoolers: Etiology and the father's role. *American Journal of Mental Deficiency, 90*, 610-617.

Goldman, S. R., & Pellegrino, J. (1987). Information processing and educational microcomputer technology: Where do we go from here? *Journal of Learning Disabilities, 20*, 144-154.

Graham, S., Harris, K. R., & Sawyer, R. (1987). Composition instruction with learning disabled students: Self-instruction strategy training. *Focus on Exceptional Children, 20*, 1-11.

Graham, S., & Harris, K. R. (1988a, April). *Improving learning disabled students' skills at generating essays: Self-instructional strategy training.* Paper presented at the AERA Annual Convention, New Orleans, LA.

Graham, S., & Harris, K. R. (1988b, April). *A component analysis of cognitive strategy instruction: Effects on learning disabled students' compositions and self-efficacy.* Paper presented at the AERA Annual Convention, New Orleans, LA.

Graham, S., & Harris, K. R. (1988c). Research and instruction in written language: Introduction to the special issue. *Exceptional Children, 54*, 495-496.

Graham, S., & Harris, K. R. (1988d). Instructional recommendations for teaching writing to exceptional students. *Exceptional Children, 54*, 506-512.

Graves, D. H. (1983). *Writing: Teachers and children at work.* Exeter, NH: Heinemann.

Gross, C. M., & Chapnik, E. B. (1987). Ergonomic training for tomorrow's office. *Training and Development Journal, 41*, 56-61.

Haggarty, R. J. (1980). Life stress, illness and social support. *Developmental Medicine and Child Neurology, 22*, 391-400.

Halpern, D. F. (1987). Analogies as critical thinking skills. In D. E. Berber, K. Pezdek, & W. P. Banks (Eds.), *Applications of cognitive psychology: Problem solving, education, and computing* (pp. 75-86). Hillsdale, NJ: Lawrence Erlbaum.

Heard, H. D., & Lake, B. (1986). The attachment dynamic in adult life. *British Journal of Psychiatry, 149*, 430-438.

Hanline, M. F., & Halvorsen, A. (1989). Parent perceptions of the integration transition process: Overcoming artificial barriers. *Exceptional Children, 55*, 487-492.

Hanzlik, J. R., & Stevenson, M. B. (1986). Interaction of mothers with their infants who are mentally retarded, retarded with cerebral palsy, or nonretarded. *American Journal of Mental Deficiency*, *90*, 513-520.

Harris, K. R., & Graham, S. (1985). Improving learning disabled students' composition skills: Self-control strategy training. *Learning Disability Quarterly*, *8*, 27-36.

Hasselbring, T. S. (1984). Using microcomputer for initiating student errors to improve spelling performance. *Computers, Reading and Language Arts*, *1*, 12-14.

Hasselbring, T. S. (1988, January). *Effective computer use in special education: What does the research tell us.* Paper presented at the Annual CEC/TAM Conference on Special Education and Technology, Baltimore.

Hasselbring, T. S., Goin, L., & Bransford, J. (1987, April). *Assessing and developing math automaticity in learning disabled students: The role of microcomputer technology.* Paper presented at the AERA Annual Convention, Washington, DC.

Hasselhorn, M., & Korkel, J. (1986). Metacognitive versus traditional reading instructions: The mediating role of domain-specific knowledge on children's text processing. *Human Learning*, *5*, 75-90.

Haynes, J., Kapinus, B., Malouf, D., & MacArthur, C. A. (1984). *Effects of computer assisted instruction on learning disabled readers' metacognition and learning of new words* (Research Report 101). College Park, MD: University of Maryland, Institute for the Study of Exceptional Children and Youth.

Helm, D. T., & Kozloff, M. A. (1986). Research on parent training: Shortcomings and remedies. *Journal of Autism and Developmental Disorders*, *16*, 1-22.

Hendrix, W. H., Steel, R. P., & Schultz, S. A. (1987). Job stress and life stress. *Journal of Social Behavior and Personality*, *2*, 291-302.

Heppner, P. P., & Krauskopf, C. J. (1987). An information-processing approach to personal problem solving. *The Counseling Psychologist*, *15*, 371-447.

Hess, R., Holloway, S., Dickson, W. P., & Price, G. (1984). Maternal variables as predictors of children's school readiness and later achievement in vocabulary and mathematics in sixth grade. *Child Development*, *55*, 1902-1912.

Hill, C. A. (1987). Social support and health: The role of affiliative need as a moderator. *Journal of Research in Personality, 21*, 127-147.

Hirst, W. (1986). Aspects of divided and selective attention. In J. LeDoux, & W. Hirst (Eds.), *Mind and Brain* (pp. 105-141). New York: Cambridge University Press.

Hirst, W., & Kalmar, D. (1987). Characterizing attentional resources. *Journal of Experimental Psychology: General, 116*, 68-81.

Hirst, W., Spelke, E., Reaves, C., Caharck, G., & Neisser, U. (1980). Dividing attention without alternation or automaticity. *Journal of Experimental Psychology: General, 109*, 98-117.

Holahan, C. J., & Moos, R. H. (1985). Life stress and health: Personality, coping, and family support in stress resistance. *Journal of Personality and Social Psychology, 49*, 739-747.

Holahan, C. J., & Moos, R. H. (1987a). Personal and contextual determinants of coping strategies. *Journal of Personality and Social Psychology, 52*, 946-955.

Holahan, C. J., & Moos, R. H. (1987b). Risk, resistance and psychological distress: A longtitudinal analysis with adults and children. *Journal of Abnormal Psychology, 96*, 3-13.

Holmes, T. H., & Rahe, R. H. (1967). The social readjustment rating scale. *Journal of Psychosomatic Research, 11*, 212-218.

Horner, C. M. (1987). Homework: A way to teach problem solving. *Academic Therapy, 22*, 239-244.

Hunt, R. A. (1985). Computers and families - An overview. *Marriage and Family Review, 8*, 11-25.

Johnson, J. H., & Sarason, I. G. (1978). Life stress, depression and anxiety: Internal-external control as a moderator variable. *Journal of Psychosomatic Research, 22*, 205-208.

Kaffman, M., Sivan-Sher, A., & Carel, C. (1981). Obstetric history of kibbutz children with minimal brain dysfunction. *Israeli Journal of Psychiatry and Related Sciences, 18*, 69-84.

Katz, E. H. (April, 1988). *Personal computers: Where to put them so children will use them.* Paper presented at the AERA Annual Convention, New Orleans, LA.

Kazak, A. E. (1987). Families of disabled children: Stress and social networks in three samples. *Journal of Abnormal Child Psychology, 15*, 137-146.

Kendall, P. C. (1977). On the efficacious use of verbal self-instructional procedures with children. *Cognitive Therapy and Research*, *1*, 331-341.

Kendall, P. C. (1985). Toward a cognitive-behavioral model of child psychopathology and a critique of related intervention. *Journal of Abnormal Child Psychology*, *13*, 357-372.

Kendall, P. C. (1987). Ahead to basics: Assessment with children and families. *Behavioral Assessment*, *9*, 321-332.

Kendall, P. C., Lerner, R. M., & Craighead, W. E. (1984). Human development and intervention in childhood psychopathology. *Child Development*, *55*, 71-82.

Kerchner, L. B., & Kistinger, B. J. (1984). Language processing/word processing: Written expression, computers, and learning disabled students. *Learning Disability Quarterly*, *7*, 329-335.

Kobasa, S. C. (1979). Stressful life events, personality and health: An inquiry into hardiness. *Journal of Personality and Social Psychology*, *37*, 1-11.

Kobasa, S. C. (1982). Commitment and coping in stress resistance among lawyers. *Journal of Personality and Social Psychology*, *42*, 168-177.

Kobasa, S. C., & Puccetti, M. C. (1983). Personality and social resources in stress resistance. *Journal of Personality and Social Psychology*, *45*, 839-850.

Kurth, R. J. (1988, April). *Process variables in writing instruction using word processing, word processing with voice synthesis and no word processing in second grade.* Paper presented at the AERA Annual Convention, New Orleans, LA.

Lamb, M. E. (1977). Father-infant and mother-infant interaction in the first year of life. *Child Development*, *48*, 167-181.

Langer, E. J. (1989). *Mindfulness*. Reading, MA: Addison-Wesley.

Lazarus, R. S., & Folkman, S. (1984). *Stress, appraisal and coping*. New York: Springer.

Lazarus, R. S., Kanner, A. D., & Folkman, S. (1980). Emotions: A cognitive-phenomenological analysis. In R. Plutchik, & H. Fellerman (Eds.), *Theories of emotions* (pp. 198-217). New York: Academic Press.

Levin, J. R. (April, 1988). *The home-school connection: A weak link in children's microcomputing efforts*. Paper presented at the AERA Annual Convention, New Orleans, LA.

Leyser, Y., Margalit, M., & Avraham, Y. (1988). Summary of research on parents with special needs children in the kibbutz. *Hachinuch Hameshutaf* (The Kibbutzim Newsletter in Education - Hebrew), *128*, 64-73.

Litt, M. D. (1988). Cognitive mediators of stressful experience: Self-efficacy and perceived control. *Cognitive Therapy and Research*, *12*, 241-260.

Lorsbach, T. C., & Worman, L. J. (1989). The development of explicit and implicit forms of memory in learning disabled children. *Contemporary Educational Psychology*, *14*, 67-76.

MacArthur, C. A. (1988a). Computers and writing instruction. *Teaching Exceptional Children*, *20*, 37-39.

MacArthur, C. A. (1988b). The impact of computers on the writing process. *Exceptional Children*, *54*, 536-542.

MacArthur, C. A., & Graham, S. (1987). Learning disabled students' composing under three methods of text production: Handwriting, word processing and dictation. *Journal of Special Education*, *21*, 22-42.

MacArthur, C. A., & Shneiderman, B. (1986). Learning disabled students' difficulties in learning to use a word processor: Implications for instruction and software evaluation. *Journal of Learning Disabilities*, *19*, 248-253.

Maddi, S. R. (1976). *Personality theories: A comparative analysis*. Homewood, IL: Dorsey.

Maddux, C. D. (1984). Using microcomputers with the learning disabled: Will the potential be realized. *Educational Computer*, *5*, 31-32.

Mahoney, M. J. (1977). A critical analysis of rational-emotive theory and therapy. *Counseling Psychologist*, *7*, 44-46.

Mahoney, M. J. (August, 1987). *Plasticity and power: Emerging emphases in theories of human change*. Presented at the APA Annual Convention, New York.

Mahoney, G. (1988). Maternal communication style with mentally retarded children. *American Journal of Mental Deficiency*, *92*, 341-348.

Mahoney, G., Finger, I., & Powel, A. (1985). Relationship of maternal behavioral style to the development of organically impaired mentally retarded infants. *American Journal of Mental Deficiency*, *90*, 296-302.

Mahoney, G., & Powel, A. (1988). Modifying parent-child interaction: Enhancing the development of handicapped children. *Journal of Special Education*, *22*, 82-96.

Malon, T. W. (1983). Guidelines for designing educational computer games. *Childhood Education, 59*, 241-247.

Margalit, M. (1982). Learning disabled children and their families: Strategies of extension and adaptation of family therapy. *Journal of Learning Disabilities, 15*, 594-595.

Margalit, M. (1984). Leisure activities of learning disabled children as a reflection of their passive life style and prolonged dependency. *Child Psychiatry and Human Development, 15*, 133-141.

Margalit, M. (1987, January). *Improving information processing for learning disabled and mentally retarded children using computer games.* Paper presented at the Annual CEC/TAM Conference on Special Education and Technology, Washington, DC.

Margalit, M., & Heiman, T. (1986). Learning disabled boys' anxiety, parental anxiety and family climate. *Journal of Clinical Child Psychology, 15*, 248-253.

Margalit, M., Leyser, Y., & Avraham, Y. (1988). Subtypes of family climate among kibbutz mothers of disabled children. *International Journal of Special Education, 3*, 101-115.

Margalit, M., Leyser, Y., & Avraham, Y. (1989). Classification and validation of family climate subtypes in the kibbutz fathers of disabled and nondisabled children. *Journal of Abnormal Child Psychology, 17*, 91-107.

Margalit, M., Leyser, Y., Avraham, Y., & Lewy-Osin, M. (1988). Social-environmental characteristics and sense of coherence in kibbutz families with disabled and nondisabled children. *European Journal of Special Education, 3*, 87-98.

Margalit, M., & Raviv, A. (1983). Mothers' perceptions of family climate in families with a mentally retarded child. *The Exceptional Child, 30*, 163-169.

Margalit, M., Rochberg, Y., & Greenberg, P. H. (December, 1988). *Technology integration in problem solving training: The family perspective.* Presented at the Annual CEC/TAM Conference on Special Education and Technology, Reno, NV.

Margalit, M., & Rot, B. Y. (in press). Strategic keyboard training and spelling improvement among children with learning disabilities and mental retardation. *Educational Psychology.*

Margalit, M., Rot, B. Y., & Greenberg, P. H. (1988). *Developing writing and spelling skills for exceptional children using computer keyboard training software.* Research report, Tel Aviv University.

Margalit, M., Shulman, S., & Stuchiner, N. (1989). Behavior disorders and mental deficiency: The family perspective. *Research in Developmental Disabilities*, *10*, 315-326.

Margalit, M., Weisel, A., & Shulman, S. (1987). The facilitation of information processing in learning disabled children using computer games. *Educational Psychology*, *7*, 47-54.

Margalit, M., Weisel, A., Heiman, T., & Shulman, S. (1988). Social skills and family climate of behavior disordered adolescents. *Behavior Disorders*, *13*, 253-262.

Mash, E., & Terdal, L. (1973). Modification of mother-child interactions: Playing with children. *Mental Retardation*, *11*, 44-49.

Mayer, R. E. (1987). Learnable aspects of problem solving: Some examples. In D. E. Berber, K. Pezdek, & W. P. Banks (Eds.), *Applications of cognitive psychology: Problem solving, education, and computing* (pp. 109-122). Hillsdale, NJ: Lawrence Erlbaum.

McCubbin, H. (1979). Integrating coping behavior in family stress theory. *Journal of Marriage and the Family*, *41*, 237-244.

McCubbin, H. I., & Patterson, J. M. (1983). The family stress process: The double ABCX model of adjustment and adaptation. *Marriage & Family Review*, *6*, 7-37.

McCutchen, D. (1988, April). *Functional automaticity in children's writing: A problem of metacognitive control.* Paper presented at the AERA Annual Convention, New Orleans, LA.

McDermott, P. A., & Watkins, M. W. (1983). Computerized vs. conventional remedial instruction for learning disabled pupils. *Journal of Special Education*, *17*, 81-88.

McGee, R., Williams, S., & Silva, P. A. (1984). Background characteristics of aggressive, hyperactive and aggressive/hyperactive boys. *Journal of the American Academy of Child Psychiatry*, *23*, 280-284.

Mitchell, R. E. (1985). The dynamics of family interaction around home video games. *Marriage and Family Review*, *8*, 121-135.

Mitchell, R. E., Billings, A. G., & Moos, R. H. (1982). Social support and well being: Implications for prevention programs. *Journal of Primary Prevention*, *3*, 77-97.

Moos, R. H. (1987a). Person-environment congruence in work, school, and health care settings. *Journal of Vocational Behavior, 31*, 231-247.

Moos, R. H. (1987b). Learning environments in context: Links between school, work, and family settings. In B. J. Fraser (Ed.), *The study of learning environments* (Vol. 2, pp. 1-16). Perth, Western Australia: Curtin University of Technology.

Moos, R. H., & Billings, A. G. (1982). Conceptualizing and measuring coping resources and processes. In L. Goldberger, & S. Breznitz (Eds.), *Handbook of stress: Theoretical and clinical aspects*. New York: Free Press.

Morocco, C. C., (1987). *Teachers, children and the magical writing machine*. Newton, MA: Educational Development Center.

Morocco, C. C., & Neuman, S. B. (1986). Word processors and the acquisition of writing strategies. *Journal of Learning Disabilities, 19*, 243-247.

Mullins, J. B. (1987). Authentic voices from parents of exceptional children. *Family Relations, 36*, 30-33.

Naisbitt, J. (1984). *Megatrends*. New York: Warner books.

Newell, A. (1980). One final word. In D. T. Tuma, & D. Reif (Eds.), *Problem solving and education: Issues in teaching and research* (pp. 175-189). Hillsdale, NJ: Lawrence Erlbaum.

Niemiec, R., & Walberg, H. J. (1987). Comparative effects of computer-assisted instruction: A synthesis of reviews. *Journal of Educational Computing Research, 3*, 19-37.

Nodine, B., Barenbaum, E., & Newcomer, P. (1985). Story composition by learning disabled, reading disabled, and normal children. *Learning Disability Quarterly, 8*, 167-179.

Norman, D. A., & Bobrow, D. B. (1975). On data-limited and resource-limited processes. *Cognitive Psychology, 7*, 44-64.

O'Leary, S. G. & Dubey, D. R. (1979). Applications of self-control procedures by children: A review. *Journal of Applied Behavior Analysis, 12*, 449-465.

Palincsar, A. S. (1986). Metacognitive strategy instruction. *Exceptional Children, 53*, 118-124.

Papert, S. (1980). *Mindstorms: Children, computers, and powerful ideas*. New York: Basic Books.

Parkerson, J. A., Lomax, R. G., Schiller, D. P., & Walberg, H. J. (1984). Exploring causal models of educational achievement. *Journal of Educational Psychology, 76*, 638-646.

Pearlin L. I., & Schooler, C. (1978). The structure of coping. *Journal of Health and Social Behavior, 19*, 2-21.

Pellegrini, A. D., Brody, G. H., & Sigel, I. G. (1985). Parents' book reading habits with their children. *Journal of Educational Psychology, 77*, 332-340.

Pellegrini, A. D., Brody, G. H., & Sigel, I. G. (1986). The effects of children's communication status and task on parents' teaching strategies. *Contemporary Educational Psychology, 11*, 1-10.

Pence, A. R. (1988). Conclusions. In A. R. Pence (Ed.), *Ecological research with children and families: From concepts to methodology* (pp. 222-226). New York: Teachers College.

Peterson, P. L. (1984). Effects of moderator variables in reducing stress outcomes in mothers of children with handicaps. *Psychosomatic Research, 28*, 337-344.

Peterson, P. L., & Wikoff, R. L. (1987). Home environment and adjustment in families with handicapped children: A canonical correlation study. *The Occupational Therapy Journal of Research, 7*, 67-82.

Pettit, G. S., Dodge, K. A., & Brown, M. M. (1988). Early family experience, social problem solving patterns and children's social competence. *Child Development, 59*, 107-120.

Pfeiffer, K., Feinberg, G., & Gelber, S. (1987). Teaching productive problem-solving attitudes. In D. E. Berber, K. Pezdek, & W. P. Banks (Eds.), *Applications of cognitive psychology: Problem solving, education, and computing* (pp. 99-122). Hillsdale, NJ: Lawrence Erlbaum.

Powell, D. R. (1988). Client characteristics and the design of community-based intervention programs. In A. R. Pence (Ed.), *Ecological research with children and families: From concepts to methodology* (pp. 122-142). New York: Teachers College.

Powell, S. (1987). Improving critical thinking: A review. *Educational Psychology, 7*, 169-185.

Pressley, M., & Levin, J. R. (1986). Elaborative learning strategies for the inefficient learner. In S. J. Ceci (Ed.), *Handbook of cognitive, social and neuropsychological aspects of learning disabilities* (pp. 175-211). Hillsdale, NJ: Lawrence Erlbaum.

Rabin, A. I., & Beit-Hallahmi, B. H. (1982). *Twenty years later: Kibbutz children grow up*. New York: Springer.

Ram, J. (1988). *Behavior and achievements of special classes' students in computer's testing and practice program (TOAM)*. Unpublished master's thesis, Tel Aviv University, Tel-Aviv, Israel.

Remp, A. M. (November, 1985). *The business education student and microcomputers: Sources of influence and information.* Paper presented at the Annual Woman Researcher Conference, Kalamazoo, MI.

Reschly, D. J. (1987). Learning characteristics of mildly handicapped students: Implications for classification, placement and programming. In M. C. Wang, M. C. Reynolds, & H. J. Walberg (Eds.), *Handbook of special education: Research and practice* (Vol. 1, pp. 35-58). New York: Pergamon Press.

Reynolds, M. C., & Lakin, K. C. (1987). Noncategorical special education: Models for research and practice. In M. C. Wang, M. C. Reynolds, & H. J. Walberg (Eds.), *Handbook of special education: Research and practice* (Vol. 1, pp. 331 - 356). New York: Pergamon Press.

Rieth, H. (1986, January). *An analysis of the instructional and contextual variables that influence the efficacy of computer-based instruction for mildly handicapped secondary school students.* Paper presented at the Special Education Technology Conference, Washington, DC.

Rodger, S. H. (1986). Parents as therapists: A responsible alternative or abrogation of responsibility? *Exceptional Child, 33*, 17-27.

Rogers, E. M. (1985). The diffusion of home computers among households in Silicon Valley. *Marriage and Family Review, 8*, 89-101.

Rokeach, M. (1968). *Beliefs, attitudes and values.* San Francisco: Jossey-Bass.

Rosegrant, T. J. (1986, April). *It does not sound right: The role of speech output as a primary form of feedback for beginning text revision.* Paper presented at the AERA Annual Convention, San Francisco, CA.

Rosenbaum, M. (1987). *Learned resourcefulness, stress, and self-regulation.* Newsletter and research report, Schwartz Research Center, Tel Aviv University, Israel.

Rosenbaum, M., & Ben-Ari, K. (1985). Learned helpfulness and learned resourcefulness: Effects of noncontingent success and failure on individuals differing in self-control skills. *Journal of Personality and Social Psychology, 48*, 198-215.

Rosenbaum, M., & Ben-Ari, K. (1986). Cognitive and personality factors in the delay of immediate gratification of hemodialysis patients. *Journal of Personality and Social Psychology, 51*, 357-364.

Roth, S., & Beck, I. (1984, April). *Research and instructional issues related to the enhancement of children's decoding skills through a microcomputer program.* Paper presented at the AERA Annual Convention, New Orleans, LA.

Russell, S. J. (1986). But what are they learning? The dilemma of using microcomputers in special education. *Learning Disability Quarterly, 9*, 100-104.

Sarason, I. G., Levine, H. M., Basham, R. B., & Sarason, B. R. (1983). Assessing social support: The social support questionnaire. *Journal of Personality and Social Psychology, 44*, 127-139.

Sarason I. G., & Sarason, B. R. (1986). Experimentally provided social support. *Journal of Personality and Social Psychology, 50*, 1222-1225.

Sarason, B. R., Sarason I. G., Hacker, T. A., & Basham, R. B. (1985). Concomitants of social support: Social skills, physical attractiveness, and gender. *Journal of Personality and Social Psychology, 49*, 469-480.

Sarason I. G., Sarason, B. R., Shearin, E. N., & Pierce, G. R. (1987). A brief measure of social support: Practical and theoretical implications. *Journal of Social and Personal Relationships, 4*, 497-510.

Schaefer, E. S., & Edgerton, M. (1985). Parent and child correlates of parental modernity. In I. E. Sigel (Ed.), *Parental belief systems* (pp. 287-318). Hillsdale, NJ: Lawrence Erlbaum.

Schiffman, G., Tobin, D., & Buchanan, B. (1982). Microcomputer instruction for the learning disabled. *Journal of Learning Disabilities, 15*, 557-559.

Schilling, R. F., Schinke, S. P., & Kirkham, M. A. (1985). Coping with a handicapped child: Differences between mothers and fathers. *Social Science Medicine, 21*, 857-863.

Schmidt, D. E., Conn, M. K., Greene, L. D., & Mesirow, K. E. (1982). Social alienation and social support. *Personality and Social Psychiatry Bulletin, 8*, 515-521.

Seitz, S., & Hoekenga, R. (1974). Modeling as a training tool for retarded children and their parents. *Mental Retardation, 12*, 28-31.

Shaw, J. S. (1982). Psychological androgyny and stressful life events. *Journal of Personality and Social Psychology, 43,* 145-153.

Short-Degraff, M. A. (1987). Commentary. *The Occupational Therapy Journal of Research, 7,* 83-92.

Sigel, I. G., & McGillicuddy-DeLisi, A. (1983). Parents as teachers of their children: A distancing behavior model. In A. D. Pellegrini, & T. Yawkey (Eds.) *The development of oral and written language in social contexts* (pp. 71-94). Norwood, NJ: Ablex.

Sitko, M. C. (December, 1988). *Application of microcomputer technology in developing writing skills in learning disabled students.* Paper presented at the Annual CEC/TAM Conference on Special Education and Technology, Reno, NA.

Sitko, M. C., & Crealock, C. M. (1986, June). *A longitudinal study of the efficacy of computer technology for improving the writing skills of mildly handicapped adolescents.* Paper presented at the Invitational Research Symposium on Special Education Technology, Washington, DC.

Smith, M. U., & Good, R. (1984). Problem solving and classical genetics: Successful versus unsuccessful performance. *Journal of Research in Science Teaching, 21,* 895-912.

Sternberg, R. J. (1985). But it is a sad tale that begins at the end: A reply to Glaser. *American Psychologist, 40,* 571-573.

Stone, A., & Michals, D. (1986). Problem solving in learning disabled children. In S. J. Ceci (Ed.), *Handbook of cognitive, social, and neuropsychological aspects of learning disabilities* (Vol. 1, pp. 291-316). Hillsdale, NJ: Lawrence Erlbaum.

Stoneman, A., Brody, G. H., & Abbott, D. (1983). In-home observations of young Down-syndrome children with their mothers and fathers. *American Journal of Mental Deficiency, 87,* 591-600.

Streibel, M. J. (1986). A critical analysis of three approaches to the use of computers in education. *Educational Communications and Technology Journal, 34,* 137-161.

Swadener, M., & Jarrett, K. (1986). Gender differences in middle grade students' actual and preferred computer use. *Educational Technology, 26,* 42-47.

Swing, R. S., Stoiber, K. C., & Peterson, P. L. (1988). Thinking skills vs. learning time: Effects of alternative

classroom-based interventions on students' mathematics problem solving. *Cognition and instruction*, *5*, 45-70.
Thomas, C., Englert, C., & Gregg, S. (1987). An analysis of errors and strategies in the expository writing of learning disabled students. *Remedial and Special Education*, *8*, 21-30.
Tognoli, J. (1980). Male friendship and intimacy across the life span. *Family Relations*, *29*, 273-279.
Torgesen, J. K. (1982). The learning disabled child as an inactive learner: Educational implications. *Topics in Learning, and Learning Disabilities*, *2*, 45-48.
Torgesen, J. K. (1984). Instructional uses of microcomputers in elementary aged mildly handicapped children. *Specialized Services in the Schools*, *1*, 37-48.
Torgesen, J. K. (1986). Computer assisted instruction with learning disabled children. In J. Torgesen, & B. Wong (Eds.), *Psychological and educational perspectives on learning disabilities* (pp. 417-435). Orlando: Academic Press.
Tremblay, R. E., Larivee, S., & Gregoire, J. C. (1985). The association between early adolescent boys' cognitive development, father attitudes and nonverbal behavior. Special Issue: Contemporary approaches to the study of families with adolescents. *Journal of Early Adolescence*, *5*, 45-58.
Trifiletti, J. K., Firth, G. H., & Amstrong, S. (1984). Microcomputer versus research rooms for learning disabled students: A preliminary investigation of the effects on math skills. *Learning Disabilities Quarterly*, *7*, 69-76.
Turkel, S. B., & Podell, D. M. (1984). Computer-assisted learning for mildly handicapped students. *Teaching Exceptional Children*, *16*, 258-262.
Turkle, S. (1984). *The second self: Computers and the human spirit*. New York: Simon and Schuster.
Unger, D. G., & Powell, D. R. (1980). Supporting families under stress: The role of social networks. *Family Relations*, *29*, 566-574.
Vacc, N. N. (1987). Word processor versus handwriting: A comparative study of writing samples produced by mildly mentally handicapped students. *Exceptional Children*, *54*, 156-165.
Vadasy, P. F., Fewell, R. R., Meyer, D. J., & Greenberg, M. T. (1985). Supporting fathers of handicapped young

children: Preliminary findings of program effects. *Analysis and Intervention in Developmental Disabilities*, *5*, 151-163.
Vaux, A. (1987). Appraisals of social support: Love, respect and involvement. *Journal of Community Psychology*, *15*, 493-502.
Vaux, A., & Athanassopulous, M. (1987). Social support appraisals and network resources. *Journal of Community Psychology*, *15*, 537-556.
Vaux, A., & Wood, J. (1987). Social support resources, behavior, and appraisals: A path analysis. *Social Behavior and Personality*, *15*, 105-109.
Vygotsky, L. S., (1978). *Mind in society: The development of higher psychological processes*. Cambridge, MA: Harvard University Press.
Werth, L. H., & Oseroff, A. B. (1987). Continual counselling intervention: Lifetime support for the family with a handicapped member. *American Journal of Family Therapy*, *15*, 333-342.
Wertheimer, M. (1985). The gestalt perspective on computer simulations of cognitive processes. *Computers in Human Behavior*, *1*, 19-33.
Westland, C. (1987). Toward a leisure-centered society: The "why", "what" and "how" of education for leisure. *European Journal of Education*, *22*, 225-232.
Wharf, B. (1988). Implementing the ecological perspective in policy and practice: Problems and prospects. In A. R. Pence (Ed.), *Ecological research with children and families: From concepts to methodology* (pp. 194-221). New York: Teachers College.
Wikler, L., Wasow, M., & Hartfield, E. (1981). Chronic sorrow revisited: Parents' vs. professionals' depiction of the adjustment of parents of mentally retarded children. *American Journal of Orthopsychiatry*, *51*, 63-70.
Wolins, I. S. (April, 1988). *The family as educator: Effects of parent-child interaction on microcomputer use*. Paper presented at the AERA Annual Convention, New Orleans, LA.
Wood, D. D., & Hollnagel, E. (1987). Mapping cognitive demands in complex problem-solving world. *International Journal of Man-Machine Studies*, *26*, 257-275.
Woodward, J., Carnine, D., & Gersten, R. (1988). Teaching problem solving through computer simulations. *American Educational Research Journal*, *25*, 72-86.

Worden, P. E.(1985, April). *Preschoolers' alphabet learning activities with their parents: Picture-books vs. personal computer software.* Paper presented at the Biennial Meeting of the Society for Research in Child Development, Toronto, Ontario, Canada.

Worden, P. E. (1986). Prose comprehension and recall in disabled learners. In S. J. Ceci (Ed.), *Handbook of cognitive, social, and neuropsychological aspects of learning disabilities* (Vol. 1, pp. 241-246). Hillsdale, NJ: Lawrence Erlbaum.

Worden, P. E., Kee, D. W., & Ingle, M. J. (1987). Parental teaching strategies with preschoolers: A comparison of mothers and fathers within different alphabet tasks. *Contemporary Educational Psychology, 12*, 95-109.

Wright, J. L. & Church, M. J. (1986). The evolution of an effective home-school microcomputer connection. *Education & Computing, 2*, 67-74.

# Author Index

# Subject Index

MIX
Papier aus verantwortungsvollen Quellen
Paper from responsible sources
FSC® C105338
FSC
www.fsc.org

If you have any concerns about our products,
you can contact us on
**ProductSafety@springernature.com**

In case Publisher is established outside the EU,
the EU authorized representative is:
**Springer Nature Customer Service Center GmbH**
**Europaplatz 3, 69115 Heidelberg, Germany**

Printed by Libri Plureos GmbH
in Hamburg, Germany